QUICK REFERENCE TO WOUND CARE

Second Edition

PAMELA BROWN, RN, BSN, CWCN, COCN
CLINICAL SPECIALIST FOR WOUND AND OSTOMY CARE
ST. JOSEPH-BAPTIST HOSPITAL
TAMPA, FLORIDA

JULIE PHELPS MALOY, ARNP, MS, CWOCN
MANAGER OF COMPREHENSIVE WOUND CENTER
CERTIFIED WOUND, OSTOMY, AND CONTINENCE NURSE; NURSE PRACTITIONER
BATTLE CREEK HEALTH CARE SYSTEM
BATTLE CREEK, MICHIGAN

JONES AND BARTLETT PUBLISHERS
Sudbury, Massachusetts
BOSTON   TORONTO   LONDON   SINGAPORE

World Headquarters
Jones and Bartlett Publishers
40 Tall Pine Drive
Sudbury, MA 01776
978-443-5000
info@jbpub.com
www.jbpub.com

Jones and Bartlett Publishers Canada
2406 Nikanna Road
Mississauga, ON L5C 2W6
CANADA

Jones and Bartlett Publishers International
Barb House, Barb Mews
London W6 7PA
UK

Cover image © Photos.com

Library of Congress Cataloging-in-Publication Data

Library of Congress Cataloging-in-Publication Data

Brown, Pamela A.
   Quick reference to wound care / Pamela Brown, Julie Phelps Maloy.—2nd ed.
     p. ; cm.
   Includes bibliographical references and index.
   ISBN 0-7637-2744-X (pbk.)
     1. Wound healing—Handbooks, manuals, etc. 2. Wounds and injuries—Treatment—Handbooks,
manuals, etc. 3. Bedsores—Nursing—Handbooks, manuals, etc.
     [DNLM: 1. Skin Ulcer—Handbooks. 2. Nursing Care—Handbooks. 3. Wounds and Injuries—Handbooks. WR
39 B879q 2004] I. Maloy, Julie Phelps. II. Title.
   RD94.B76 2004
   617.1'06—dc22

                                                                     2004013531

Acquisitions Editor: Kevin Sullivan
Production Director: Amy Rose
Production Assistant: Caroline Senay
Associate Marketing Manager: Emily Ekle
Editorial Assistant: Amy Sibley
Manufacturing Buyer: Amy Bacus
Cover Design: Timothy Dziewit
Composition: Viewtistic, Inc.
Technical Artist: George Nichols
Printing and Binding: Malloy, Inc.
Cover Printing: Malloy, Inc.

Printed in the United States of America
09 08 07 06 05   10 9 8 7 6 5 4 3 2 1

CONTENTS

PART I—ASSESSMENT AND DOCUMENTATION

PART II—BASICS OF WOUND MANAGEMENT

PART III—WOUND TYPES COMMONLY
SEEN BY HEALTH CARE PROFESSIONALS

PART IV—ISSUES SPECIFIC TO HOME HEALTH
AND SKILLED NURSING FACILITIES

CONTRIBUTORS

Pamela Brown, RN, BSN, CWCN, COCN
Clinical Specialist for Wound and Ostomy Care
St. Joseph-Baptist Hospital
Tampa, Florida

Christopher A. Morrison, MD, CSW
Medical Director & President
Nautilus Health Care Group
Tierra Verde, Florida

Julie Phelps Maloy, ARNP, MS, CWOCN
Manager of Comprehensive Wound Center
Certified Wound, Ostomy, and Continence Nurse; Nurse Practitioner
Battle Creek Health Care System
Battle Creek, Michigan

Susan V. McGovern, ARNP, MS
Quality Improvement Coordinator
FMQAI: Florida ESRD Network

Donna Oddo, RN, BSN, CWOCN
Clinical Specialist for Wound, Ostomy, and Continence Care
Independent Community Hospital
New Port Richey, Florida

Ben Peirce, RN, CWOCN
Manager of Wound Care
Gentiva Health Services
Melville, New York

ACKNOWLEDGMENTS

A special thank you to my husband, Warren Clark, for his patience and support; and to the nurses and caregivers who work hard to provide compassionate healing care. This book is for them.

—Pamela Brown

I would like to acknowledge my appreciation for Pam Brown for her words of encouragement coupled with a wonderful sense of humor throughout our book revision process. I appreciate the support of my husband and family as night after night I would vanish into my office. In addition, I have great admiration for the many nurses who fearlessly ask questions as they strive toward improving the quality of the care provided to those who have wounds.

—Julie Maloy

INTRODUCTION

Historically, wound care treatment was anecdotal. There were few scientifically based treatments available. With the advent of the concept of moist wound healing, things began to change. Today there are many different treatments available that are based on sound scientific research. Effective, scientifically based wound care is now recognized as a key factor in helping patients heal more quickly and move more economically through the health care system. Changes in Medicare and managed care are demanding more cost-effective plans of treatment. A huge industry is building up around the heightened interest in wound care.

Even with major advances in wound care in the last 30 years, wound management in many settings may not be scientifically based. Wound healing can be slow and sporadic. For optimal healing to occur, a plan must be developed that will incorporate wound etiology, appropriate assessment skills, principles of wound healing, scientifically based treatments, and prevention measures. The plan needs to include appropriate goals for wound healing and reevaluation of the process at regular intervals.

The main purpose of this book is to provide health care professionals with information that is easy to use, so they can provide optimal wound care in the most cost-effective manner. This is a nuts-and-bolts book that covers the basics in wound care from A to Z. The most common wound types are illustrated with color photographs. There are numerous exhibits to aid clinicians in assessment, documentation, and day-to-day treatment of wounds.

Part I includes a chapter written by a physician. This chapter gives a concise description of what a physician needs to know when developing a plan of care for a patient with a wound. This section also includes a chapter with step-by-step instructions for accurate assessment and documentation of wounds. Accurate assessment and documentation are important for communication between medical professionals and directly affects reimbursement issues.

Part II addresses the normal healing process, basics of wound management, and topical treatments. Using the information in these chapters, a clinician can assess the patient, develop an individualized care plan, determine the appropriate healing goals, and match the dressing to the wound.

Part III includes chapters on the major wound types that are most commonly seen by health care professionals. Each chapter focuses on a specific wound type. The etiology of the wound types, treatments, and prevention are included. Teaching guides, case studies, and tips from experience punctuate the main points covered in this section.

Part IV addresses issues specific to home health care and extended care facilities. Criteria for admission, reimbursement issues, and documentation are discussed for each setting.

The authors are enterostomal therapy nurses with over 30 years combined experience in home care and extended care settings. This book is written as a quick reference. Contributors include a physician who specializes in wound care, the manager of wound care for a national home health agency, and nurses who specialize in treating persons affected by wounds. For more in-depth information on topics covered in this book, or for wound types not addressed, the reader should refer to more comprehensive wound care resources.

PART I

Assessment and Documentation

CHAPTER 1

Initial Wound Assessment and Communication

Christopher A. Morrison

Thanks to advancements in technology, our ability to communicate with one another is unprecedented. However, it seems that communication among health care providers regarding patient care is at an all time low. Health care is trying to cope with increased patient volumes, decreased revenue, and the burden of documentation. As medicine continues to subspecialize, providers must communicate with greater precision. This is certainly true for wound care. Very often the prescribing physician relies on communication with the treating nurse to help determine an appropriate wound care treatment plan.

Communication needs to cover the diagnosis and treatment of the physical and mental characteristics of a patient. This combination of physical and mental assessment is especially important for those with nonhealing wounds. Popular belief holds that advanced technologies have improved our healing outcomes. Actually, the strongest gains in wound healing have come from sharpened assessment and aggressive treatment of the underlying factors that can impede healing. That means a thorough assessment is a must when a patient is admitted to your agency or facility. As the treating nurse, your job is to take an accurate history and to examine the patient. Then you need to describe your findings, document them in the medical record, and communicate your findings with the treating physician. All the nurses caring for the patient need to follow through by assessing wound progress accurately and communicating effectively with the rest of the treating team. This is important not only for the care of the patient but also because of today's medical malpractice climate.

MEDICAL HISTORY

The patient's medical history is key to understanding possible physiological influences on wound healing. This information can help identify local and systemic risk factors that impede wound healing. Some of these include:

- Tissue oxygen perfusion
- Edema
- Bacterial bioburden
- Pressure, shear, friction
- Nutritional status
- Central circulatory dysfunction including congestive heart failure and chronic obstructive pulmonary disease
- Chronic illness including diabetes mellitus, renal insufficiency, and malignancy
- Dermatological abnormalities including skin cancer, dermatitis, previous radiation, and scarring
- Inflammatory or autoimmune disorders including vasculitis, rheumatoid arthritis, scleroderma, and lupus
- Coagulation disorders
- Immunosuppression including corticosteroids and chemotherapy
- Age
- Physiologic and psychological stress

WOUND HISTORY

The patient's wound healing history can yield helpful information for implementing the wound care plan:

- Does the patient have a history of previous nonhealing wounds?
- How long has the patient had the current wound?
- What caused or may have caused the current wound?
- Were there past treatments used on the wound? Were they successful?
- Who was the treating physician?
- Was any diagnostic testing undertaken (noninvasive vascular studies, radiographs, other imaging studies, or cultures)?

Wound Assessment

Accurate assessment of the wound is crucial for determining appropriate topical and systemic therapies that might aid in healing.

- Record length, width, and depth of the wound.

- Note depth and location of any undermining or tunneling. Use the face of a clock for orientation with 12 o'clock being toward the head of the patient and 6 o'clock toward the feet. Undermining is defined as space that extends under the skin or superficial tissue and usually involves a larger area of the border of the wound (i.e., 1.5 cm undermining from 3 o'clock to 7 o'clock). A tunnel is a narrow passageway extending from the open wound under intact tissue (i.e., tunneling 3 cm at 5 o'clock). A tunnel has an end and is dead space. Don't confuse a tunnel with a fistula. A fistula is an abnormal passage connecting two or more structures or spaces. It can connect one body cavity or hollow organ to another or to the skin.
- Describe the condition of the wound tissue. Mention the presence, color, and percentage of healthy granulation tissue, fibrous tissue or slough, necrotic tissue, eschar, or gangrene.
- Report any exposed tendon, ligament, muscle, or bone, as well as its color and overall appearance.
- Describe the characteristics of the wound drainage. Note the amount (large, moderate, minimal) and type of fluid (serous, serosanguinous, bloody, purulent).
- Inspect the condition of the periwound area, noting erythema, warmth, maceration, fluctuance, scarring, and dermatitis.
- If the wound involves a lower extremity, thorough physical examination can give immediate insight into the underlying etiologies of nonhealing. Note skin color and quality (normal, thin, shiny, dry, scaly, erythematous, brawny, etc.). Note presence of edema (1+ to 4+) and any weeping or drainage from the leg. Record the temperature of the legs, feet, and toes (warm, cool, cold). Note the presence or absence of hair on the legs, feet, and toes. Check for capillary refill at the toenail beds (i.e., less than 3 sec.). Assess the femoral, popliteal, dorsalis pedis, and posterior tibial arteries.
- Because pain is now considered the fifth vital sign, ask the patient to assess the pain on a scale of 1–10. Pain provides important information and can significantly impact the patient's quality of life and ability to heal. An extremely painful wound can signify an inflammatory condition (pyoderma gangrenosum, vasculitis) or infection. Ischemic ulcers can also be very painful and may indicate the presence of underlying peripheral vascular disease. As pain is usually subjective, it is best to have the patient rate his or her pain on a scale of 1 to 10 (10 being the worst pain they have ever felt).

Risk Factors

To be as successful as possible in healing chronic wounds, you must be proactive. You must assess the patient as a whole, including underlying risk factors that may play a part in nonhealing. This comprehensive assessment aids healing outcomes and can help prevent further problems.

- Flexion contractures of the extremities that place excessive axial loading force on the wound or other bony prominence should be identified. To decrease the likelihood of poor outcomes, the recommendation of appropriate off-loading devices is important.
- Note the type of mattress, cushion, and any other off-loading pressure devices that the patient is using. Also, communicate where (and in which position) the patient spends his or her time.
- A nutritional assessment, if available, should be communicated.
- Note any known history of noncompliance or inability to follow instructions.

The wound assessment report to the attending physician should be a concise two- to three-minute summary. It should contain wound characteristics and descriptions, and all other pertinent patient information. With this type of initial wound assessment and communication, the patient will benefit from a team health care approach. Appropriate initial treatment increases likelihood for a positive outcome. Exhibit 1-1 is a sample wound report prepared for a physician.

Exhibit 1–1 Sample Wound Report

WOUND REPORT SHEET   Medical Record #:_____

Date: _____   Patient Name: _____   Date of Birth: _____

Diagnoses: <u>UTI, IDDM, CHF</u>_____

Wound Location: <u>Stage III Pressure Ulcer in the coccygeal area</u>_____
(Use additional page for additional wounds)

Pressure Ulcer: Stage _____<u>III</u>____; or Partial Thickness _____ Full Thickness _____

Size: <u>3.5cm</u> Lx <u>5.3cm</u> Wx <u>2.0cm</u> D; undermining/tunneling _____ cms. located @ _____ o'clock

Wound Bed: <u>45</u> % Red, <u>55</u> % Yellow, _____ % Black, _____ Other (Describe) _____

Wound Margins: <u>Macerated and Open</u>____ (Closed, reddened, warm, tender, macerated, denuded)

Exudate Amount: <u>Dressing saturated at change</u> Type: ___<u>serous</u>___, Odor noted (Y/N): ____<u>No</u>____

Pain Assessment: <u>Medicated for dressing change; pain level 6 prior to medication</u>_____

Current Treatment: <u>Wet to dry dressing changes BID</u>_____

_____

Impressions: <u>Wet to dry dressing changes are painful. Periwound is macerated from excessive moisture.</u>
<u>Increase of approx. 10% amt. of healthy red tissue within the last week. Yellow tissue has decreased.</u>____

_____

_____

Recommendations: <u>Stop wet to dry BID changes. Begin wound care daily with calcium alginate to control</u>
<u>the exudate, decrease maceration. Apply cover dressing.</u>_____

_____

Name of person making report (Please Print): <u>Jane Doe RN</u>_____

Signature of person making report: _____<u>Jane Doe RN</u>_____ Phone Number: __<u>818-888-8888</u>__

Physician: Please write your orders for wound care below, and contact ___<u>HH Supervisor</u>___
at Phone: _____ **Fax:** _____
Physician: Please print & sign your name below:

Doctor's Name: _____   **Signature:** _____

(See next page for blank Wound Report Sheet.)

Exhibit 1–2 Sample Wound Report

WOUND REPORT SHEET   Medical Record #:_____

Date: _____   Patient Name: _____   Date of Birth: _____

Diagnosis: _____

Wound Location:_____
(Use additional page for additional wounds)

Pressure Ulcer: Stage _____; or Partial Thickness _____ Full Thickness _____

Size: _____ Lx _____ Wx _____ D; undermining/tunneling _____ cms. located @ _____ o'clock

Wound Bed: _____ % Red, _____ % Yellow, _____ % Black, _____ Other (Describe) _____

Wound Margins: _____ (Closed, reddened, warm, tender, macerated, denuded)

Exudate Amount: _____ Type: _____, Odor noted (Y/N): _____

Pain Assessment: _____

Current Treatment: _____
_____

Impressions: _____
_____
_____
_____

Recommendations: _____
_____
_____

Name of person making report (Please Print): _____

Signature of person making report: _____ Phone Number: _____

Physician: Please write your orders for wound care below, and
contact _____ **at Phone:** _____ **Fax:** _____
Physician: Please print & sign your name below:

Doctor's Name: _____ Signature: _____

CHAPTER 2

Assessment and Documentation for Wounds: A Step-by-Step Process

Pamela Brown

Wound care begins with a careful and thorough assessment. The clinician should determine the etiology of the wound and any factors that could impact the healing process. Ongoing assessment should be done at regular intervals, ideally weekly, to determine healing progress. Consistency in wound assessment is important. The wound should be evaluated with the patient in the same position each time, and preferably by the same clinician. Photography or tracings can be used as documentation tools and can provide helpful information. Accurate documentation enables critical evaluation of the wound healing progress. It can also directly impact reimbursement and help protect clinicians against litigation.

WOUND CLASSIFICATION

Skin, the body's largest organ, is divided into two layers: the epidermis and the dermis. Underneath these lie subcutaneous tissue, fascia, muscle, and bone. The classification of a wound is determined by the number of layers it penetrates.

1. Partial-thickness wounds involve the epidermis and extend into, but not through, the dermis. Examples are tape burns, sunburns, blisters (unless blood filled, which could indicate deeper tissue damage), some skin tears, and Stage II pressure ulcers (Figures 2–1 and 2–2; Color Plates 1 and 2).
2. Full-thickness wounds involve a subcutaneous layer or extend into muscle or bone. Examples are deep leg ulcers, deep burns, and Stage III or Stage IV pressure ulcers.

WOUND STAGING

If the wound is a pressure ulcer, you must stage it. It is important to remember that staging is inappropriate until nonviable tissue is removed from the wound bed. Until necrotic tissue is removed and the wound bed

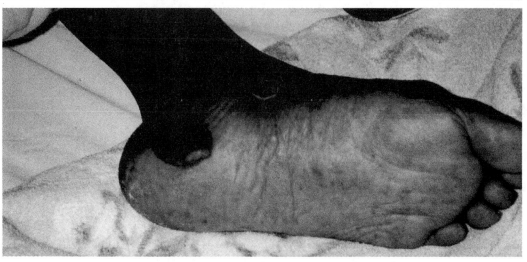

Figure 2–1 Intact Purple Heel Blister.
Clinical Objectives:
(1) Protect
(2) Relieve pressure
See Color Plate 1.

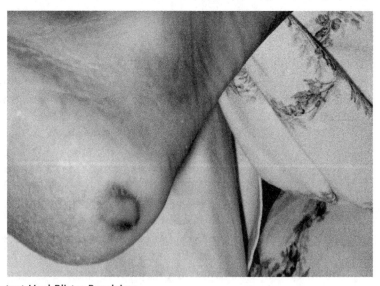

Figure 2–2 Intact Heel Blister Resolving.
Clinical Objectives:
(1) Protect
(2) Relieve pressure
See Color Plate 2.

is visible, the wound is unstageable (Bergstrom et al., 1994, 18). Once the wound stage is identified, the wound should not be backstaged. As a Stage IV pressure ulcer heals, it is a healing Stage IV. Once it is closed, it is a healed Stage IV. (See Exhibit 6–1, page 96, for National Pressure Ulcer Advising Panel's Staging of Pressure Ulcers.)

WOUND LOCATION AND DIMENSIONS

The wound location should be precisely identified. Use directional terms like right or left, medial or distal, and the correct anatomic location. A body drawing can be used (Figure 2–3).

The dimensions of the wound should be measured and recorded weekly. Measure the length, width, and depth in centimeters. A disposable tape measure can be used.

Measure the length at the longest point on the wound surface, measured head to toe.

Measure the width at the widest point on the wound surface, measured side to side.

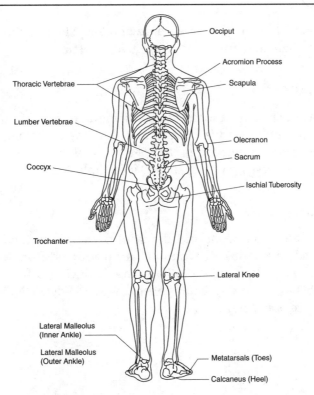

Figure 2–3 Common Locations for Chronic Wounds.

To determine a wound's depth, insert a sterile, cotton-tipped applicator into the deepest part of the wound bed, grasp the applicator at skin level, and then measure the applicator from its tip to your fingers.

Wound tunneling (Color Plate 7) or undermining (Color Plate 13) is measured by inserting a cotton-tipped applicator to measure depth in centimeters. Describe the location using the face of a clock, with 12 o'clock at the patient's head, and 6 o'clock at the patient's feet. Always work in a clockwise direction when documenting the deepest sizes of tunneling or undermining. *Example:* 2 cm of undermining from 2 o'clock to 6 o'clock.

WOUND BED

Note the status of the wound bed. Document necrotic tissue, fibrin slough, and red granulation tissue. Quantifying the percentage of tissue involved can help paint a picture of the wound bed and facilitate assessment and documentation of changes in the wound bed. *Example:* The wound bed is 50 percent black eschar, 25 percent fibrin slough, and 25 percent red granulation tissue.

WOUND ODOR

Note the presence or absence of odor. When you detect an odor, note its strength and any identifying characteristics.

WOUND DRAINAGE

Describe any exudate, including the amount, color, and characteristics such as serous, purulent, or viscous. *Example:* Is the old dressing dry? Is it 25 percent, 50 percent, or 100 percent saturated? How long has it been since the dressing was changed? (See Table 2–1.)

WOUND MARGINS

Assess the extent and depth of undermining and the condition of wound edges. Are the wound edges macerated from too much moisture or rolled under? Are they sharp and distinct or diffuse and irregular? Is epithelial tissue visible around the wound edges? Note the presence or absence of induration.

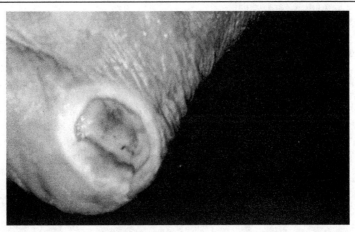

Figure 2–4 Heel Ulcer with Yellow Slough. Periwound skin macerated due to inappropriate topical treatment.

Clinical Objectives:

(1) Clean

(2) Remove necrotic tissue

(3) Manage exudate

(4) Relieve pressure

See Color Plate 3.

TIPS   A plastic sandwich bag can be used for tracing the wound. Place the bag on the wound, and trace the outline of the wound with a permanent, fine-tip marker. Add location markers such as head, feet, and anatomical location. Throw away the side that was touching the wound, and place the clean side with the tracing in the chart.

PERIWOUND SKIN

Assess color, induration, warmth, and edema of the skin around the wound. Redness of the surrounding skin can be indicative of unrelieved pressure. Irritation of the surrounding skin can result from exposure to feces or urine, a reaction to the dressing or tape, or inappropriate removal of dressing or tape. Redness, tenderness, warmth, and swelling are classical clinical signs of infection.

Table 2–1 Wound Exudate Characteristics

Exudate Type	Color	Consistency	Significance
Sanguineous/bloody	Red	Thin, watery	Indicates new blood vessel growth or disruption of blood vessels
Serosanguineous	Light red to pink	Thin, watery	Normal during inflammatory and proliferative phases of healing
Serous	Clear, light color	Thin, watery	Normal during inflammatory and proliferative phases of healing
Seropurulent	Cloudy, yellow to tan	Thin, watery	May be first signal of impending wound infection
Purulent/pus	Yellow, tan, or green	Thick, opaque	Signals wound infection; may be associated with odor

PAIN

Note presence or absence of pain in the wound or periwound area. Use your agency's guidelines for assessing pain.

REFERENCE

Bergstrom, N. et al. 1994. *Treatment of pressure ulcers.* Clinical Practice Guideline No. 15. AHCPR Publication No. 95-0652. Rockville, MD: U.S. Department of Health and Human Services. Public Health Services, Agency for Health Care Policy and Research.

BIBLIOGRAPHY

Cooper, D. 2000. Assessment, measurement, and evaluation: Their pivotal roles in wound healing. In *Acute and chronic wounds: Nursing management,* ed. R. Bryant, 51–81. St. Louis, MO: Mosby.

Sussman, C. 1998. Assessment of the skin and wound measurement. In *Wound care: A collaborative practice manual for physical therapists and nurses,* eds. C. Sussman and B. M. Bates-Jensen, 49–102. Gaithersburg, MD: Aspen Publishers, Inc.

Van Rijswijk, L. 1997. Wound assessment and documentation. In *Chronic wound care: A clinical source book for healthcare professionals,* 2d ed., eds. D. Krasner and D. Kane, 16–27. Wayne, PA: Health Management Publications.

PART II

Basics of Wound Management

CHAPTER 3

Normal Healing Process

Pamela Brown

To best understand the normal healing process, the clinician needs to know the structure of the skin (Figure 3–1).

STRUCTURES OF THE SKIN

The skin is the largest organ of the body. It consists of two layers: epidermis and dermis.

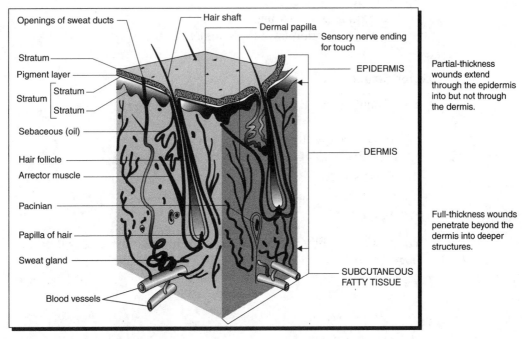

Figure 3–1 Anatomy of the Skin.

Epidermis

The epidermis is the outermost layer of skin. It varies in thickness, but is usually around 0.1 mm thick with five layers of squamous cells.

Functions

- protection from ultraviolet light and outside contamination
- sensations
- temperature control
- prevention of dehydration
- Vitamin D production
- may indicate the emotional state of the patient

Dermis

The dermis is connected to the epidermis by a basement membrane.

Functions

- hair production (hair follicles)
- sensation (nerve endings)
- supplier nourishment (removes waste via capillaries)
- provides elasticity (elastin)
- strength support (collagen)
- sweat production (sweat glands)

Deeper Structures

The subcutaneous tissue is called the hypodermis.

- located below dermis
- provides insulation and protection for organs
- stores energy

WOUND HEALING PROCESS

The wound healing process is divided into two categories (See Table 3–1 page 19).

1. Partial-thickness wounds penetrate the epidermis and may extend into the dermis. They heal by epithelialization; that is, the epithelial cells migrate from the wound edges and any remaining hair follicles to resurface the wound. These wounds are usually moist and painful because of the loss of epidermal covering and exposure of nerve endings.

2. Full-thickness wounds extend beyond the dermis into the subcutaneous tissue. They can also involve muscle, tendon, or bone and heal by filling with granulation tissue, contraction, and epithelialization from the wound edges. The healing process is one of granulation tissue formation and contraction.

Acute wounds progress through a predictable series of events that result in a healed wound. This process can be described as a cascade of events with healing phases that overlap. The final result is a healed wound. In contrast, chronic nonhealing wounds fail to proceed through an orderly and timely healing process.

Table 3–2, page 20, gives an overview of the normal healing process for full-thickness wounds.

Table 3–1 Partial-Thickness and Full-Thickness Skin Loss

Thickness of Skin Loss	Definition	Clinical Examples
Partial-thickness skin loss	Extends through the epidermis, into but not through the dermis	Skin tears, abrasions, tape damage, blisters, perineal dermatitis from incontinence; heals by epidermal resurfacing or epithelialization
Full-thickness skin loss	Extends through the epidermis and the dermis, extending into subcutaneous fat and deeper structures	Donor sites, venous ulcers, arterial/ischemic wounds; surgical wounds; heals by granulation tissue formation and contraction

Table 3–2 Normal Healing Process for Full-Thickness Wounds

	Inflammatory Phase* (1 to 4 days postinjury)	Proliferation Phase* (4 to 20 days postinjury)	Maturation Phase* (21 days to 2 years postinjury)
Main function	Initial healing cascade; removes debris and prepares for new tissue	Deposition of connective tissue and collagen cross-linking	Strengthening and reorganizing of collagen fibers
Clinical observations	Pain, redness, swelling, heat Serous or serosanguineous drainage	Extracellular matrix, commonly called granulation tissue, fills the wound bed with newly formed collagen and blood vessels. The appearance is beefy red. Epithelial cells migrate across the wound surface from wound margins.	Shrinking, thinning, paling of scar
Physiologic actions	Bacteria are killed. Cellular debris is removed. The wound is prepared for tissue regeneration: • Platelets cause blood clotting. • Vasoconstriction and vasodilation direct blood to where it's needed. • Leukocytes and macrophages engulf and kill bacteria.	Macrophages continue to kill bacteria. Fibroblasts deposit collagen to fill the wound bed. New blood vessels extend into the area (angiogenesis). Myofibroblasts cause the wound to contract.	New tissue continues to grow and develop, and the scar is strengthened. Collagen fibers reorganize and remodel, and wound contraction continues.
Tips	If the patient is immunocompromised, inflammation will be suppressed. Risk of infection will increase, and healing can be delayed.	A change from beefy red to dusky pink (with or without an increase in drainage) can be a sign of infection.	Even when the wound is completely healed, only about 80% of tensile strength of normal skin is regained. The patient is at risk for recurrent breakdown.

*These phases overlap and occur as a cascade of healing events. For more detailed information on a cellular level, refer to the bibliography at the end of this chapter.

BIBLIOGRAPHY

Cooper, D. 1990. The physiology of wound healing: An overview. In *Chronic wound care: A clinical source book for healthcare professionals*, ed. D. Krasner, 1–11. King of Prussia, PA: Health Management Publications.

Haimowitz, J., and Margolis, D. 1997. Moist wound healing. *Chronic wound care: A clinical source book for healthcare professionals*, 2nd ed., eds. D. Krasner and D. Kane, 49–56. Wayne, PA: Health Management Publications.

Sussman, C. 1998. Wound healing biology and chronic wound healing. In *Wound care: A collaborative practice manual for physical therapists and nurses*, eds. C. Sussman and B. M. Bates-Jensen, 31–45. Gaithersburg, MD: Aspen Publishers, Inc.

Waldrop, J. & Doughty, D. 2000. Wound healing physiology. In R. A. Bryant (Ed.) *Acute & Chronic Wounds: Nursing Management* (2nd ed.) (17–39). St. Louis, MO: Mosby, Inc.

CHAPTER 4

Basics of Wound Management

Pamela Brown

Wound healing is a complex process involving many factors. When developing a wound healing treatment plan, the clinician should assess the entire patient. The plan should address causative factors and factors that are known to impede the healing process. Dressings should protect the wound, provide a moist environment, and prevent maceration of wound edges. The goal is to create an environment that promotes wound healing and supports the body in healing itself. It is imperative to reevaluate the healing progress at regular intervals. If a wound shows no healing progress in two to four weeks, reevaluate the patient and the wound treatment plan. Report your findings to the physician.

CAUSATIVE FACTORS

Reduce or eliminate factors that cause wounds. Failure to reduce or eliminate the cause can result in a nonhealing wound despite appropriate systemic and topical therapy.

Pressure

A pressure ulcer is an area of local tissue trauma usually developing where soft tissue is compressed between a bony prominence and any external surface for prolonged time periods. A pressure ulcer is a sign of local tissue necrosis and death.

Friction

Friction is the resistance generated between two objects as they are moved in opposite directions. *Example:* Skin can be denuded during repositioning.

Shear

Shear occurs when two surfaces are being moved in opposite directions and they do not slide freely across each other. This causes deformities, kinking, or tearing of vessels in deep tissue. *Example:* When the head of the bed is up and the patient slides down in bed, the skin and superficial fascia can remain fixed against the bed linen, while the deep fascia and skeleton slide down toward the foot of the bed, causing deep tissue damage.

Circulatory Impairment

Compromised circulation, such as peripheral vascular disease and chronic obstructive pulmonary disease, affect healing at a cellular level. Tissue repair is compromised in the absence of adequate blood supply and/or oxygenation.

Neuropathy

Loss of sensation puts the patient at risk for mechanical, chemical, and thermal trauma. This occurs as a complication of prolonged glucose elevation.

Moisture

Moisture, urine, and feces can cause maceration and overhydration of the epidermis. The skin tissue becomes less tolerant to pressure force.

SYSTEMIC SUPPORT

Provide systemic support for wound healing.

Nutrition and Hydration

Failure to address poor nutritional status will result in a nonhealing wound despite appropriate topical therapy. If a patient is at risk, a clinical dietitian should assess the patient as part of a multidisciplinary approach to wound management (Exhibits 4–1, page 25, and 4–2, page 27). Look for

- patients weighing less than 80 percent of ideal body weight
- an involuntary weight loss of 10 percent or greater
- serum albumin (a measure of protein available for healing) less than 3.5
- total lymphocyte count less than $1800/mm^3$

Exhibit 4–1 Skin Integrity and Wound Healing: The Role of Nutrition

It has long been recognized but unappreciated that impaired nutritional status and inadequate dietary intake are risk factors for development of pressure ulcers. A well-balanced diet with adequate carbohydrate, protein, fat, water, vitamins, and minerals is necessary to maintain skin integrity.

Calories, protein, water, vitamin C, and zinc are often emphasized to promote wound healing. However, adequate intake of these nutrients or any nutrient alone does not facilitate healing. Sufficient calories plus all essential nutrients are required.

CALORIES

The body's first priority is adequate energy. When the total amount of calories is too low, protein from both the diet and the patient's muscle stores is used as an energy source, the patient loses weight, and adipose tissue as well as lean body mass is lost.

Every wound patient's calorie needs are different. The caloric goal for patients with wounds is to prevent weight loss from occurring. In underweight patients, a slow steady weight gain will increase the speed of wound healing. The three major nutrients—carbohydrate, protein, and fat—provide calories. Carbohydrates and fats are the preferred energy source for a healing wound.

PROTEIN

Dietary protein is needed for tissue maintenance and repair. Protein depletion impairs wound healing by preventing a desirable wound bed from forming. Repletion of calorie and protein status in undernourished patients is associated with shorter time to heal and improved wound strength. In general, a wound patient's daily dietary protein needs (expressed as grams of protein) can be estimated by dividing the patient's weight in half. For example, a patient who weighs 100 pounds would need approximately 50 g of protein daily to heal wounds. Too high a protein intake will increase fluid needs, and wound healing will be reduced if fluid needs are not met.

WATER

Water is an especially important nutrient for patients with wounds. Dehydration is a risk factor for development of wounds, and the water needs of patients with Stages III and IV pressure ulcers are very high. A good rule of thumb is to be sure that all patients receive a minimum of 1 milliliter (ml) of water for every kilocalorie fed, or about 15 ml of water per pound of body weight per day. Wound patients need at least 2000–2500 ml of water a day (2 quarts or more).

Water and other household beverages are adequate sources of water in most cases and can be given orally or by feeding tube. These fluids, however, are not adequate to replace the fluid and electrolyte losses that accompany vomiting, diarrhea, or other sources of gastrointestinal fluid losses. In these cases, a rehydration solution, such as Equalyte® (Ross Products Division of Abbott Laboratories), that is specifically designed to match and replace these losses is needed.

continues

Exhibit 4–1 continued

VITAMIN C

Because nutritional deficiency has been associated with impaired wound healing, supplemental intake of vitamins and minerals is often thought to be important for wound healing. Although not appropriate for all patients, vitamin and mineral supplements are probably most beneficial for patients with a history of poor intake who are therefore likely to have limited nutrient stores. A general one-a-day type vitamin and mineral supplement equal to 100 percent of the Reference Daily Intake (RDI) for vitamins and minerals is prudent for patients with wounds.

Vitamin C is essential in collagen synthesis. Collagen and fibroblasts compose the basis for the structure of a new healing wound bed. A deficiency of vitamin C prolongs healing time, decreases wound strength, and contributes to decreased resistance to infection. There is no evidence, however, that human wound healing is improved by providing doses of vitamin C many times greater than the RDI of 60 milligrams (mg) per day. It is reasonable to increase vitamin C intake through consumption of fruits, vegetables, and juices for persons with extensive wounds who may rapidly exhaust their body reserves and for those with a history of poor intake.

ZINC

Zinc deficiency can occur through wound drainage or excessive gastrointestinal fluid losses or can be due to long-term low dietary intake. Chronic, severe zinc deficiency results in abnormal function of white blood cells and lymphocytes, increased susceptibility to infection, and delayed wound healing. Large amounts of dietary zinc, however, interfere with copper metabolism and are not advisable. The amount of zinc in a multiple vitamin/mineral supplement is generally adequate. It is much more preferable and safer to provide the RDI for zinc (12–15 mg/day) through a one-a-day type multiple vitamin and mineral supplement than to provide individual zinc supplementation at very high levels (such as zinc sulfate 200–300 mg daily or three times daily).

Proper hydration is needed to promote blood flow to affected areas (Exhibit 4–3, page 28).

Diabetes

Wound healing is impaired in patients with diabetes, and they have an increased incidence of infection. Their plan of care should include strict control of blood glucose levels.

Steroid Administration

Steroids are known to inhibit epithelial proliferation and to exert powerful anti-inflammatory effects. Vitamin A can partially counteract the effect of steroids.

Exhibit 4–2 Suggested Diet for Wound Healing

- *Calories (energy)*—provide enough calories to prevent weight loss, promote wound healing, and prevent infection; 30–35 calories per kilogram (kg) body weight per day.

- *Protein*—adequate for positive nitrogen balance and to promote new cell development; 1.2–2 g of protein per kg of body weight per day.

- *Fluid*—30 ml per kg body weight per day; adjust per individual need.

- *Vitamin/minerals*

  - Vitamin C helps make collagen, promotes healing, and helps build resistance to infection.

  - Vitamin A helps make new skin cells.

  - Zinc promotes wound healing and improves immunity.

  - Iron helps carry oxygen to nourish the cells.

Note: Vitamin/mineral supplementation is often recommended if the oral diet is inadequate. If deficiencies are confirmed or suspected, a multivitamin may be used. Due to toxicity and nutrient interactions, multivitamins should not be used in high doses and should only be used if ordered by the physician. See suggested Nutrient–Rich Foods for Wound Healing page 43 and High-Calorie/High-Protein Ideas page 45 at the end of this chapter.

Immunosuppression

Any disease process or medication that suppresses the immune system can delay wound healing.

Aging

The aging process produces many changes in the skin that can impede the healing process. It is important to optimize healing and to eliminate any correctable impediments to healing. Optimal systemic and topical support will enhance the healing process.

Obesity and Wound Healing

There are multiple issues to consider for the patient who is morbidly obese. Frequently, these patients have numerous co-morbidities compli-

Exhibit 4–3 Signs and Symptoms of Dehydration

- If the client/resident is able to drink independently, keep water or other beverages at bedside so that they are easily accessible and in a container that can be handled easily.

- If the client/resident doesn't initiate drinking, offer water each time the client/resident is turned (every two hours).

Look for:

- dry skin
- cracked lips
- thirst (may be diminished in the elderly)
- fever
- loss of appetite
- nausea
- dizziness
- increased confusion
- increase in pulse
- constipation (recent diarrhea can explain the dehydrated state, whereas constipation is a common occurrence when dehydration exists)
- concentrated urine

cating their care and their wound care. Some of these co-morbidities can include: diabetes, cardiovascular disease, hypertension, and social and psychological stress.

In the home environment, it may be necessary not only to include special equipment, but also to have the environment evaluated to see if the additional equipment can be used safely and effectively. Special consideration must also be given to prevent injury to the caregivers.

In the hospital and nursing home environment, standard equipment weight limits may not provide safety for the patient. Weight limits must be considered for all of the equipment used in the care of the obese patient. Special equipment with weight loads over 500–600 pounds may be required. This can include beds, side rails, lifts, wheelchairs, stretchers, walkers, and toilet facilities.

Issues to consider include:

- Nutrition
- Mobility

- Wound considerations
- Pain management

Developing protocols to implement when a morbidly obese patient is admitted to service can provide direction for decision making and care planning. This can be invaluable in preventing complications. For more detailed information, refer to the resource list below and bibliography (at the end of this chapter).

Resources:

- www.hill-rom.com
- www.kci.com
- www.sizewiserentals.com

PRINCIPLES OF TOPICAL THERAPY

The goal of topical therapy is to create an environment that supports the healing process.

Remove Necrotic Tissue

Necrotic tissue can be removed in several ways (Figure 4–1; Color Plate 4). See Table 4–1, page 31, Debridement Time Frames.

1. mechanical debridement
   - wet-to-dry gauze moistened with normal saline. This is a non-selective method and may remove healthy tissue as well as necrotic tissue. This method of debridement is used less today than in the past because safer, more effective treatments are available. Another wound care treatment should be used once the wound bed is cleaned of necrotic tissue.
   - whirlpool—for removal of thick exudate, slough, or necrotic tissue. It should be discontinued when the wound bed is clear of necrotic tissue.
   - wound irrigation. Safe and effective ulcer irrigation pressures range from 4 to 15 psi (pounds per square inch).
2. enzymatic debridement—ointments used on necrotic tissue to clean the wound bed (see Enzymatic Debriders in Chapter 5).
3. sharp debridement—surgical debridement of necrotic tissue. Use clean, dry dressing for 8 to 24 hours after sharp debridement associated with bleeding. Then resume moist dressings.

4. autolytic debridement—breakdown of necrotic tissue by the body's wound fluids, which contain natural enzymes. A moisture-retentive dressing can be used for autolytic debridement. Do not use on infected wounds (Figure 4–2; Color Plate 5).

- transparent film dressings
- hydrogel dressings
- hydrocolloid dressings

See Debridement Choices for chronic wounds at the end of this chapter, page 49.

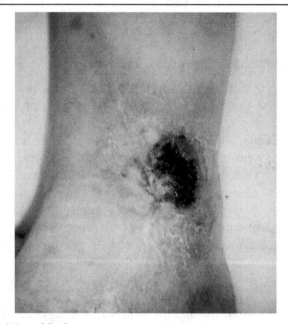

Figure 4–1 Eschar on Wound Bed.
Clinical Objectives:
(1) Remove eschar
(2) Provide moist wound environment
(3) Manage exudate
See Color Plate 4.

Table 4-1 Debridement Time Frames

Necrotic Tissue Type	Debridement Choice	Expected Outcomes	Time Frame Guide	Notes
Eschar	Autolysis	1. Eschar nonadherent to wound edges 2. Necrotic tissue lifting from wound edges 3. Necrotic tissue soft and soggy 4. Color change from black/brown to yellow/tan	14 days	Depending on type of dressing used for autolysis, may proceed at more rapid rate
Eschar	Enzymatic preparations	1. Eschar nonadherent to wound edges 2. Necrotic tissue lifting from wound edges 3. Necrotic tissue soft and soggy 4. Color change from black/brown to yellow/tan 5. Change from eschar to slough	14 days	Requires compliance with dressing changes in order to be effective
Eschar	Sharp	1. Removal/elimination of eschar if done one time or significant change in amount and adherence if sequential	Immediate if one time, 7 days if sequential	If sequential sharp debridement used in conjunction with enzymatic preparation or autolysis, may expect clean wound base in 7 days
Slough or fibrin	Autolysis or enzymatic preparations	1. Necrotic tissue lifting from wound base 2. Necrotic tissue stringy or mucinous 3. Tissue color yellow or white 4. Change in amount of wound covered—gradual decrease to wound predominantly clean	14 days	Will require moderate amount of exudate absorption and protection of surrounding tissues from maceration
Slough or fibrin	Sharp	1. Removal/elimination of necrotic slough if done one time or significant change in amount and adherence if sequential	Immediate if one time, 7 days if sequential	If sequential sharp debridement used in conjunction with enzymatic preparation or autolysis, may expect clean wound base in 7 days

---

TIP FOR EFFECTIVE IRRIGATION   A 35-ml syringe and a 19-gauge needle or angio-cath can be used to irrigate the wound with normal saline. This will provide safe and effective irrigation of 8 psi.

Identify and Eliminate Infection

All wounds are colonized with bacteria. Healing may be impaired if bacterial levels exceed 100,000 per gram of tissue or if the patient has osteomyelitis. Colonization may be minimized through effective wound

---

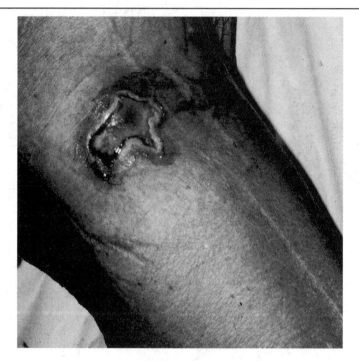

Figure 4–2 Autolytic Debridement in Progress: Slough Wound Base.
Clinical Objectives:
(1) Clean
(2) Remove slough
(3) Keep moist
(4) Relieve pressure
See Color Plate 5.

---

cleansing and debridement. Proper cleansing of the wound is one of the most effective and most often overlooked ways to keep the bacterial level down in a wound. Use minimal mechanical force when cleaning a wound with gauze, cloth, or sponges. Traumatized wounds are more susceptible to infection and are slower to heal. Healthy tissue can be damaged. Normal saline is the preferred cleansing agent because it will not harm healing tissue, and it adequately cleans most wounds. If the pressure is too high, it can damage healing tissue. If irrigation pressures are too low, they will not cleanse the wound properly. Safe and effective irrigation pressures of 4 to 15 psi can be obtained using a 19-gauge needle or angiocath with a 35-ml syringe. Pressurized saline designed for wound cleansing is also available (Table 4–3, page 34, and Exhibit 4–4, page 35). Signs and symptoms of infection include

- a wound that does not progress toward healing despite optimal care for two to four weeks
- increased drainage with or without foul odor
- purulent drainage (thick green or yellow)
- redness or warmth around wound
- cellulitis of surrounding tissue
- pain

Treat Localized Infection

For localized signs of infection, or wounds that do not show progress toward healing after two to four weeks of optimum care, a two-week trial of silver composite or topical antibiotic should be considered. *Do not use topical antiseptics such as povidone iodine, iodophor, Dakins Solution, hydrogen peroxide, or acetic acid to decrease bacteria in wound tissue.* Numerous studies have shown these antiseptics to be toxic to healing tissue. If no improvement is seen, quantitative bacterial cultures may be ordered. Swab cultures are of questionable value because they detect only the surface contaminants and may not truly reflect the organism(s) causing the infection. However, they may be ordered by the physician if clinical signs of infection are present.

TIP FOR SWAB CULTURE   First, cleanse the wound with normal saline. Swab the wound bed using a Z technique. Pressure is applied to the swab to cause tissue/fluid to be absorbed in the swab. Place the swab in the appropriate container immediately and transport it to the lab.

Table 4-3 Comparison of Wound Characteristics in Inflamed and Infected Wounds

Wound Characteristic	Inflamed Wounds	Infected Wounds
Erythema (redness or purple-gray color)	Usually presents with well-defined borders. Not as intense in color. May be seen as skin discoloration in dark-skinned persons, such as a purple or gray hue to the skin or a deepening of normal ethnic color.	Edges of erythema or skin discoloration may be diffuse and indistinct. May present as very intense erythema or discoloration with well-demarcated and distinct borders. Red stripes streaking up or down from the area indicate infection.
Elevated temperature	Usually noted as increase in temperature at wound site and surrounding tissues.	Systemic fever (may not be present in older adult populations).
Exudate: odor	Any odor present may be due to necrotic tissue in the wound, solubization of necrotic tissue, or the type of wound therapy in use, not necessarily infection.	Specific odors are related to some bacterial organisms, such as the sweet smell of *Pseudomonas* or the ammonia odor associated with *Proteus*.
Exudate: amount	Usually minimal; if injury is recent, you should see a gradual decrease in exudate amount over 3–5 days.	Usually moderate to large amounts; if injury is recent, you will not see a decrease in exudate amount—the amount remains high or increases.
Exudate: character	Bleeding and serosanguineous to serous. Variable.	Serous and seropurulent to purulent.
Pain		Pain is persistent and continues for an unusual amount of time. Take wound etiology and subjective nature of pain into account when assessment is performed.
Edema and induration	May be slight swelling or firmness at wound edge.	May indicate infection if edema and indurations are localized and accompanied by warmth.

Exhibit 4–4 Proper Procedures for Cleaning Wounds

SHALLOW WOUND CLEANSING PROCEDURE

Supplies

- clean, shallow container
- saltwater solution or wound cleanser solution
- gauze
- catch basin
- wound dressing

Procedure

1. Follow universal precautions regarding handwashing, gloving, and protection from splashing.

2. Warm the saltwater solution or wound cleanser solution to lukewarm. Test the temperature with your elbow.

3. Pour the amount of solution you expect to use into a clean, shallow container. Then the balance of the solution will remain clean.

4. Moisten a pad of clean gauze dressing (bandage) with the solution in the clean, shallow container.

5. Place the catch basin under the wound edge to collect the fluid.

6. Work in a circular pattern, starting at the center of the wound, to gently cleanse the wound with the moistened gauze. Work outward toward the edge of the wound and surrounding skin. Remove any pus or loose tissue with the gauze pad. Do not press hard or scrub because this will damage the tissue and slow healing. Do not return to the wound center after cleansing. This will recontaminate the wound.

7. Discard the moist gauze and any unused solution in the container.

8. Apply the prescribed dressing (bandage) as directed.

Helpful hint: Keep the patient and the room warm while cleansing the wound. The patient will be more comfortable. Cooling will slow the healing of the wound.

DEEP WOUND CLEANSING PROCEDURE

Deep wounds often have tunnels that run under the skin. Pus and dead tissue trapped in these tunnels are sources for infection. These tunnels can be cleansed by using a syringe filled with saltwater solution to flush them.

continues

Exhibit 4–4 continued

SUPPLIES

- 35-ml size syringe
- saltwater solution
- gauze
- catch basin
- towels
- wound dressing

PROCEDURE

1. Follow universal precautions regarding handwashing, gloving, and protection from splashing.

2. Warm the saltwater solution to lukewarm. Test the temperature with your elbow.

3. Fill a 35-ml syringe with warm saltwater solution.

4. Place a catch basin and clean towels under the wound edge to collect the fluid.

5. Insert the tip end of the syringe into the tunnel and squirt fluid into the tunnel. Put in the entire amount of the solution that is in the syringe. Repeat three times or until the fluid that comes out is clear, whichever occurs last.

6. Following the running out of the solution, gently massage the tissues with your fingers to express extra fluid.

7. After the wound is cleansed, loosely pack it with dressing materials as prescribed. This will help to prevent infection from traveling up the tunnel.

8. The dirty fluid collected in the basin should be flushed down the toilet.

Helpful hint: Keep the patient and the room warm while cleansing the wound. This will make the patient more comfortable. Cooling will slow the healing of the sore.

Treat Systemic Infection

For systemic signs of infection, such as fever, chills, weakness, or increased heart rate, the patient should be evaluated immediately for bacteremia, sepsis, advancing cellulitis, or osteomyelitis and treated with the appropriate antibiotic.

Pack Dead Space

Open cavities provide a collection space for wound exudate, which can be a medium for bacterial growth and abscess formation. Open cavities, including sinus tracts, should be loosely packed to absorb drainage and prevent superficial wound closure over a fluid-filled defect (Figures 4–3 and 4–4; Color Plates 6 and 7).

Absorb Excess Exudate

Large amounts of exudate can macerate periwound skin.

Maintain Moist Wound Surface

A moist wound surface facilitates wound healing. Choose a dressing that keeps the surrounding intact skin dry while keeping the wound bed moist.

Protect against Heat and Cold

Epidermal migration is enhanced when normal body temperature is maintained.

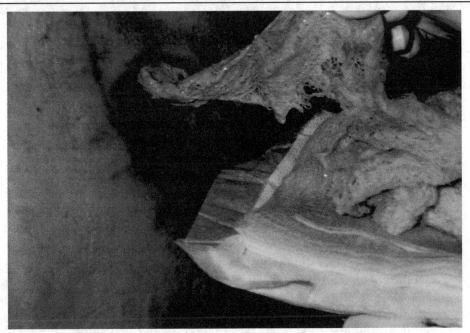

Figure 4–3 Chest Tube Site with Copious Purulent Drainage on Gauze Packing.
Clinical Objectives:
(1) Clean
(2) Manage exudate
(3) Loosely pack dead space
(4) Culture if appropriate
See Color Plate 6.

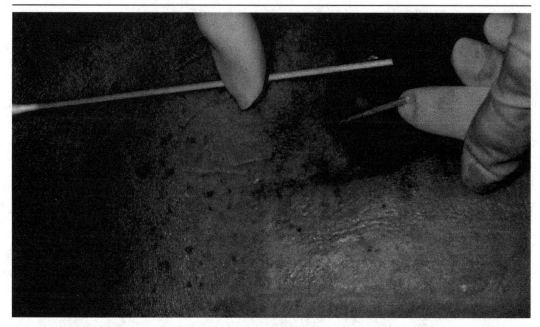

Figure 4–4 Chest Tube Site (Same as Previous Picture) with Large Tunnel.
Clinical Objectives:
(1) Clean
(2) Pack wound loosely
(3) Manage exudate
See Color Plate 7.

Protect the Healing Wound

Healing tissue is very fragile, and a dressing should protect it from trauma and invasion.

Pain

All patients should be assessed for pain. If they are experiencing pain, the etiology must be determined. Is the pain related to the disease process or the treatment? Once the etiology is determined, interventions can be planned, such as covering the wound, adjusting support services, and repositioning. Analgesics should be provided as needed.

CLEAN, NO-TOUCH WOUND CARE IN THE HOME

Handwashing is the single most important means of preventing the spread of infection.

The Agency for Health Care Policy and Research Guidelines, recently renamed the Agency for Healthcare Research and Quality, for the treatment of pressure ulcers states: "Clean dressings, as opposed to sterile ones, are recommended for home use until research demonstrates otherwise. This recommendation is in keeping with principles regarding nosocomial infections, and with past success of clean urinary catheterization in the home setting, and takes into account the expense of sterile dressings and the dexterity required to apply them (Bergstrom et al., 1994, 65). The no-touch technique can be used for dressing changes." This technique is a method of changing surface dressings without touching the wound or the surface of any dressing that might be in contact with the wound. In conjunction with this technique, a clean field is prepared, clean gloves are worn to remove the dressing, and a new pair of gloves is donned to apply the new dressing. Steps are included to prevent direct contamination of material and supplies. Many agencies use a no-touch technique. Follow your agency's policy.

WOUND CARE SOLUTIONS YOU CAN MIX AT HOME

Normal saline is a safe, effective, non-cytotoxic solution that is used for wound cleansing.

Dakin's Solution and acetic acid should not be routinely used in wound care. Studies have shown that they are cytoxic to wounds. However, there may be circumstances when they can be used for a short period of time, and a physician orders them. These solutions can be prepared in the home. Use your agency's policy for clean verses sterile preparation. Below is a chart for making these solutions in the home. Label all containers. The solution is stable for 24 hours from date of preparation.

Solution	Ingredients
0.9% normal saline	4 cups sterile water,* 2 tsp salt (iodized or noniodized table salt)
.025% acetic acid	5 cups sterile water, 4 tb white distilled vinegar
Dakin's Solution	
Full strength (0.50)	1 pint sterile water, 50 ml bleach
Half strength (0.25)	1 pint sterile water, 25 ml bleach
Quarter strength (0.125)	1 pint sterile water, 12.5 ml bleach

*To prepare sterile water, boil water for 20 minutes.

CASE STUDY

Mrs. Jones is an 84-year-old woman who lives with her husband in a single-family home. She has a diagnosis of dementia. Her husband is the primary caregiver and is 86 years old. Four months ago her condition deteriorated, and her husband was no longer able to get her out of bed. He began using diapers to manage incontinence and fed her small meals five or six times a day. He hired a caregiver who came four hours two mornings a week.

After three months in bed, Mrs. Jones developed a pressure ulcer on her sacrum. For one month, Mr. Jones provided wound care using home remedies. To his untrained eye, the wound was not getting better. He notified the physician, and arrangements were made for a home visit by the doctor. After the visit, the doctor ordered wound care of gauze moistened with normal saline twice a day and a home health evaluation.

The RN case manager assessed the wound as a Stage III pressure sore with enough depth to need packing. The wound measured 3 centimeters (cm) long, 2 cm wide, and 1.5 cm deep. The wound bed was 100 percent red granulation tissue. There was a moderate amount of serous drainage. The wound edges were intact. There were no signs or symptoms of infection. The RN recommended the following plan:

1. lab work to assess Mrs. Jones's nutritional status (Her serum albumin was 3.5.)
2. a Foley catheter to manage urinary incontinence
3. bed pads instead of diapers
4. a hospital bed with a standard mattress, and an overlay for pressure reduction (After one month, if no improvement is seen, the support service can be upgraded to a Group 2 replacement mattress.)
5. skilled nurses three times a week to teach the caregiver how to care for a bedbound, total care patient. The teaching guide, Exhibit 6–5, page 113, will be used to plan Mrs. Jones's individualized care.

After one month, the wound was improving, and Mr. Jones had been instructed in his wife's care. Skilled nurses were then reduced to once a week to assess wound healing progress and to change the Foley catheter monthly. The Foley will be discontinued when the wound is healed.

TIP   With limited nursing visits available, it is imperative to have a plan of care in place as soon as possible. Caregivers must be included in the plan so that they will be able to provide the care when nursing is not available.

REFERENCE

Bergstrom, N. et al. 1994. *Treatment of pressure ulcers*. Clinical Practice Guideline No. 15. AHCPR Publication No. 95-0652. Rockville, MD: U.S. Department of Health and Human Services. Public Health Services, Agency for Health Care Policy and Research.

BIBLIOGRAPHY

Alvarez, O. et al. 1990. Principles of moist wound healing : Indications for chronic wounds. In *Chronic wound care: A clinical source book for health care professionals*, ed. D. Krasner, 266–281. King of Prussia, PA: Health Management Publications.

Doughty, D. B. 1992. Principles of wound healing and wound management. In *Acute and chronic wounds: Nursing management*, ed. R. Bryant, 1–25. St. Louis, MO: Mosby-Year Book.

Gallagher, S., and Gates, J. (2003). Obesity, panniculitis, pannicalectomy, and wound care: Understanding the challenges. *Journal of Wound, Ostomy and Continence Nursing* 30(6), 334–341.

Krasner, D., and Kane, D., eds. 1997. *Chronic wound care*, 2d ed. Wayne, PA: Health Management Publications.

Mulder, D. et al. 1998. *Clinicians' pocket guide to chronic wound repair*. Springhouse, PA: Springhouse Corp.

Murphy, K., and Gallagher, S. 2001. Options in practice: Care of an obese patient with an ulcer. *Journal of Wound, Ostomy and Continence Nursing*, 28(3). 171–176.

Rolstad, B. S. et al. 2000. Principles of wound healing. In *Acute and chronic wounds: Nursing management*, ed. R. Bryant, 85–112. St. Louis, MO: Mosby, Inc.

Sussman, C., and Bates-Jensen, B., eds. 1998. *Wound care: A collaborative practice manual for physical therapists and nurses*. Gaithersburg, MD: Aspen Publishers, Inc.

Suggested Nutrient-Rich Foods for Wound Healing

FOODS RICH IN PROTEIN
- beef
- chicken
- pork
- turkey
- fish
- beans
- milk
- cheese
- ice cream
- peanut butter
- eggs
- nuts
- cottage cheese
- yogurt

FOODS RICH IN VITAMIN C
- oranges
- orange juice
- grapefruit
- broccoli
- lemons
- cantaloupe
- green pepper
- strawberries
- kale
- cabbage
- tomatoes
- turnip greens
- juices with vitamin C added

FOODS RICH IN VITAMIN A
- liver
- egg yolks
- broccoli
- kale
- greens
- apricots
- cantaloupe
- sweet potatoes
- whole milk
- fortified skim or low-fat milk
- carrots
- spinach

FOODS RICH IN ZINC
- shellfish
- oatmeal
- rice
- eggs

continues

**FOODS RICH IN ZINC
(continued)**

- nuts
- organ meats (liver, heart, gizzard)
- dried beans and peas
- yogurt

FOODS RICH IN IRON

- liver
- beef
- pork
- beans
- spinach
- peanuts
- sardines
- tuna
- dried fruit
- egg yolks
- oysters
- enriched bread/cereals with iron
- raisins

Combine iron-rich foods or supplement with vitamin C–rich foods for best absorption.

High-Calorie/High-Protein Ideas

GOALS

- to eat enough calories to prevent protein from being used as energy instead of for tissue building
- to provide enough calories and protein to reach and maintain goal weight

SUGGESTIONS

Cheese

Melt on sandwiches, meats, fish, vegetables, and eggs. Grate in sauces, casseroles, mashed potatoes, rice, pastas, and breads. Stuff into vegetables and meatloaf. Spread cream cheese on sandwiches, sliced fruit, and crackers. Mix cottage cheese in pastas, gelatins, pancake batter, and egg dishes.

Whole Milk/Cream

Add or substitute for water in food preparation. Serve cream sauces on vegetables, eggs, pastas, or rice. Pour cream on cereals, fruits, desserts. Top desserts, fruits, molded salads, and hot beverages with whipped cream.

Powdered Milk

Blend 1 cup powdered milk into 1 quart whole milk to make it higher in protein and calories. Add powder to meatloaf, casseroles, sauces, cream soups, and shakes.

Ice Cream/Yogurt

Spread between cookies, cake slices, or graham crackers. Blend into shakes, sodas. Add to cereals, fruits, gelatins, desserts, and pies. Top with fruit, nuts, syrups, sauces, whipped cream, and nut butters.

Eggs

Top salads, vegetables, casseroles, soups, stews, pastas, and potatoes with chopped, hard-cooked eggs. Add pasteurized egg substitute into mashed potatoes, vegetable purées, shakes, and malts. Do not consume raw eggs.

Nuts/Nut Butter

Spread nut butters on sandwiches, toast, muffins, crackers, fruit slices, pancakes, and waffles. Use as a dip for raw vegetables and fruit. Add to meatloaf, cookies, bread, muffins, vegetables, and salads. Blend nut butters with milk drinks, or swirl through ice cream and yogurt. Top cookies or cakes with nut butters. Serve nuts as snacks. Roll bananas in chopped nuts.

Meat/Fish

Use in omelets, soufflés, quiches, sandwich fillings, and poultry stuffing. Add small pieces to vegetable salads, casseroles, soups, stuffed baked potatoes, and biscuit ingredients. Wrap in pie crust or biscuit dough as turnovers.

Peas/Beans

Add cooked dry peas and beans or tofu to soups, pastas, casseroles, and meat or milk-based dishes. Mash with cheese and milk. Add textured vegetable protein to burgers, meatloaf, spaghetti sauce, casseroles, and sandwich filling.

ADDITIONAL TIPS

You don't always have to eat a lot, but try to eat often. Try using liquid nutritional supplements between meals to help increase your nutritional intake. (They are available in grocery stores and drug stores.)

To increase calories, drink fruit juice instead of water. Double or triple the portion sizes of added fats and oils (butter, margarine, cream cheese, sour cream, avocado).

SNACKS

Try to eat six times a day, or every two to three hours. Watch the clock! Eat, even if you are not hungry.

250-CALORIE SNACKS

- 8 buttery style crackers, 1 oz cheddar cheese, or 1 tb peanut butter
- ½ sandwich: 1 slice bread, 2 oz cheese or meat, 1 tsp mayonnaise
- quesadilla: 1 tortilla, 2 oz cheese, salsa
- whole apple (sliced) with 2 tb peanut butter
- 1 cup pudding or fruit yogurt
- 1 slice pizza with extra cheese
- 1 cup whole milk mixed with ⅓ cup dry skim milk powder
- 8-oz can liquid nutritional supplement providing 1 calorie per ml (250 calories/8-oz serving)

350-CALORIE SNACKS

- 10 buttery style crackers, 2 oz cheddar cheese, or 2 tb peanut butter
- ½ sandwich: 1 slice bread, 2 oz meat or cheese, 2 tsp mayonnaise, 1 slice avocado
- 1 tortilla, 2 oz cheese, salsa, with 1 cup orange juice
- whole banana with 2 tb peanut butter

- 1 envelope instant breakfast made with whole milk
- shake made with 1 cup whole milk and ½ cup ice cream
- 1 carton regular yogurt (not low-fat), with ⅓ cup granola or trail mix
- 8-oz can liquid nutritional supplement providing 1.5 calories per ml (350 calories/8-oz serving)

Debridement Choices
for Chronic Wounds

Wound Type	Tissue Type	Consistency	Adherence	Amount of Debris	Debridement Choices	Rationale and Notes
Pressure sores	Black/brown eschar	Hard	Firmly adherent, attached to all edges and base of wound	75%–100% of wound covered	1. *Autolytic*—best choice is transparent film dressing. May use hydrocolloid or hydrogel; score eschar with scalpel for more rapid results. 2. *Enzymatic ointment with secondary dressing*—must score eschar with scalpel.	1. Transparent film dressings trap fluid at the wound surface with no absorptive capabilities, providing for more rapid hydration of the eschar and facilitating autolysis. Hydrocolloid/hydrogel dressings have an absorptive capacity and may require more time for autolysis. 2. Enzymatic ointments effective against collagen and protein may be most effective.
	Black/brown eschar or Yellow/tan slough	Soft, stringy Soft, soggy	Adherent, attached to wound base; may or may not be attached to wound edges	50%–100% of wound covered	1. *Autolytic*—best choices are hydrocolloids and hydrogels; composite dressings may also be beneficial. 2. *Enzymatic ointment with secondary dressing.*	1. Hydrocolloids and hydrogels provide for absorption of mild to moderate amounts of exudate while maintaining a wound environment to facilitate autolysis.

Wound Type	Tissue Type	Consistency	Adherence	Debris	Debridement Choices	Rationale and Notes
Pressure sores (continued)					3. *Sharp, sequential, or one time* — may be used alone or in conjunction with any of the above methods.	2. Enzymatic ointments effective against collagen and protein may be most effective. May need to protect intact skin from enzyme and excess exudate.
	Yellow/tan slough	Soft, stringy	Adherent, attached to wound base, may or may not be attached to wound edges or loosely adherent to wound base	Less than 50% of wound covered	1. *Autolytic*—best choices are hydrocolloids and hydrogels. 2. *Enzymatic ointment with secondary dressing.* 3. *Sharp, sequential, or one time* — may be used alone or in conjunction with any of the above methods.	1. Hydrocolloids and hydrogels provide for absorption of mild to moderate amounts of exudate while maintaining a moist wound environment to facilitate autolysis. 2. Enzymatic ointments effective against collagen and protein may be most effective. May need to protect intact skin from enzyme and excess exudate.

Wound Type	Tissue Type	Consistency	Adherence	Amount of Debris	Debridement Choices	Rationale and Notes
Pressure sores (continued)	Yellow slough	Mucinous	Loosely adherent to wound base, clumps scattered throughout wound	50%–100% of wound covered	1. *Autolytic*—best choices are hydrocolloids and hydrogels. 2. *Enzymatic ointment with secondary dressing.*	1. Hydrocolloids and hydrogels provide for absorption of mild to moderate amounts of exudate while maintaining a moist wound environment to facilitate autolysis. 2. Enzymatic ointments effective against collagen and protein may be most effective. May need to protect intact skin from enzyme and excess exudate. Should be discontinued when wound is predominantly clean.
Venous disease ulcers	Black/brown eschar	Hard	Firmly adherent, attached to all edges and base of wound	50%–100% of wound covered	1. *Autolytic*—best choices are hydrocolloids and hydrogels. 2. *Enzymatic ointment with secondary dressing.*	1. Hydrocolloids and hydrogel dressings have absorptive capacity, which helps prevent maceration of surrounding tissues and promotes autolysis.

Wound Type	Tissue Type	Consistency	Adherence	Amount of Debris	Debridement Choices	Rationale and Notes
Venous disease ulcers (continued)						2. Enzymatic ointments effective against fibrin may be most effective.
	Yellow slough	Soft, soggy, or fibrinous	Firmly adherent, attached to all edges and base of wound	50%–100% of wound covered	1. *Autolytic*—best choice are hydrocolloids and hydrogels. 2. *Enzymatic ointment with secondary dressing.* 3. *Sharp, sequential, or one time*—may be used alone or in conjunction with any of the above methods.	1. Hydrocolloids and hydrogel dressings have absorptive capacity, which helps prevent maceration of surrounding tissues and promotes autolysis. 2. Enzymatic ointments effective against fibrin may be most effective. May need to protect intact skin from enzyme and excess exudate. Should be discontinued when wound is predominantly clean.

Wound Type	Tissue Type	Consistency	Adherence	Amount of Debris	Debridement Choices	Rationale and Notes
Venous disease ulcers (continued)	Yellow slough	Fibrinous or mucinous	Loosely adherent Clumps scattered throughout wound	Any amount of wound covered	1. *Autolytic*—best choices are hydrocolloids and hydrogels. 2. *Enzymatic ointment with secondary dressing.*	1. Hydrocolloids and hydrogel dressings have absorptive capacity, which helps prevent maceration of surrounding tissues and promotes autolysis. 2. Enzymatic ointments effective against fibrin may be most effective. May need to protect intact skin from enzyme and excess exudate. Should be discontinued when wound is predominantly clean.
Neurotrophic/ diabetic ulcers	White/gray	Hard	Hyperkeratosis, callus formation at wound edges	Involves all/partial wound edges	1. *Sharp, sequential, or one time—* saucerization or callus removal. 2. *Autolytic*—best choices are hydrocolloids and hydrogels.	1. Saucerization may be required at each dressing change. 2. Hydrocolloids and hydrogels soften the callus formation, and this may facilitate dressing removal.

Extreme caution should be taken when caring for patients with ischemic ulcers on lower extremities. See Chapter 7.

CHAPTER 5

Wound Treatments

Donna Oddo

There is no "magic" dressing. Wound dressings are but one component of the formula necessary to heal a patient's wound. It is always necessary to assess the whole patient, treat the underlying cause of the wound, and support wound healing with careful attention to all factors that can delay healing.

Selection of an appropriate wound dressings can be challenging. Health care and wound care are undergoing constant change, and nurses must educate themselves on the principles of wound healing as well as new products. The most common topical treatments are presented in this chapter. The examples provided are not inclusive of all available products, and no endorsement is intended or implied.

To determine the appropriate topical treatment, the clinician must assess the wound bed, wound drainage, depth of tissue damage, presence of infection, and the type and location of the wound. These characteristics will help determine the overall goal of treatment (Table 5–1 on page 56, and Figure 5–2 on page 73 will help the clinician choose the appropriate wound care. Exhibit 5–3 on page 79 gives guidelines for teaching wound care to patients and caregivers).

TIP In the home setting, all topical treatments require a physician's order. (See Exhibit 5–1, page 57, for "Nuggets from Experience." See Appendix 5–A, page 83, to contact manufacturers for more information on products.)

TRADITIONAL GAUZE DRESSINGS

Gauze dressings may be nonadherent, woven, or nonwoven. They are moderately absorptive, cost-effective, and easily available. They can be combined with topical agents or other types of dressings. They can cover or fill a wound. They can be loosely packed into tunneling wounds

continues on page 58

Table 5–1 Topical Treatment Options

Wound Type (Color/Exudate)	Goal	Wound Depth	
		Superficial	Cavity
Black/low exudate	Rehydrate and loosen eschar. Enhance autolytic debridement.	Hydrogels Hydrocolloids Transparent films Enzymatic debriders	
Yellow/high exudate	Remove slough and absorb exudate.	Hydrocolloids Alginates Enzymes Hydrofiber Foam	Hydrogels Moist packing gauze Enzymes Alginates Hydrofiber Collagen
Yellow/low exudate	Remove slough, absorb exudate, and maintain a moist environment.	Hydrogels Sheet hydrogels Hydrocolloids Transparent film	Hydrogels Impregnated gauze Moist packing gauze Alginates Enzymes
Red/high exudate	Maintain moist environment, absorb exudate, and promote granulation and epithelialization.	Foam Alginates Hydrofibers	Alginates Hydrofiber Moist packing gauze
Red/low exudate	Maintain moist environment and promote granulation and epithelialization.	Hydrocolloids Foam Sheet hydrogels Transparent films	Hydrogels Moist packing gauze
Pink/low exudate	Maintain moist environment, and protect and insulate.	Foams Transparent films Hydrocolloids (thin) Nonadherent dressing	
Red, unbroken skin	Prevent skin breakdown	Hydrocolloids Transparent films	

Exhibit 5–1 Nuggets from Experience

MACERATION

Maceration is softening of tissue due to excessive moisture. Wound edges become white and soft. When maceration occurs around wound edges, skin barrier cream or wipes should be applied. If maceration continues to occur, consider a more absorptive dressing or increase the frequency of dressing changes until drainage decreases.

HYPERGRANULATION

When granulation tissue proliferates and overlaps the wound bed, epithelialization cannot occur. Consider a more absorptive dressing to manage the hypergranulation tissue. If this is not effective, paint the tissue daily with betadine to suppress the hypergranulation and allow the epithelial cells to migrate over the granulation tissue. Discontinue the betadine when the hypergranulation tissue is resolved. Silver nitrate can be used to cauterize the hypergranulation tissue and allow epithelialization to occur. Repeat applications may be necessary (Figure 5–1; Color Plate 8).

SHARPS DEBRIDEMENT

When bleeding occurs after sharps debridement, appropriate care is a clean, dry dressing for 8 to 24 hours. Then resume moist wound care.

MALIGNANCY

Be aware that unusual chronic wounds and wounds that fail to heal after adequate therapy may require a biopsy to rule out malignancy.

ROLLED EDGES

Full-thickness chronic wounds may have thick, rolled edges. Epithelial cells have migrated down and around the wound edges. For the wound to complete the healing process, silver nitrate can be applied to the wound edges. Another choice is to allow the wound edges to become macerated. The goal is to break down the rolled edges so that epithelialization of the wound surface can occur.

HEEL ULCERS WITH DRY ESCHAR

The Agency for Health Care Policy and Research Guidelines state that "heel ulcers with dry eschar need not be debrided if they do not have edema, erythema, fluctuance, or drainage. Assess these wounds daily to monitor for pressure ulcer complications" (Bergstrom et al., 1994, 49).

OCCLUSIVE DRESSINGS

Do not use occlusive dressings such as hydrocolloids on infected wounds or wounds with potential for anaerobic infection. Do not use on deep cavity wounds or wounds with undermining or sinus tracts. Discontinue the dressing if undermining or sinus tracts develop.

continues

Exhibit 5–1 continued

DRY GANGRENE

Do not attempt wound care of dry gangrene. If the physician is aware of the situation and a conservative course of treatment is indicated, keep the site clean, dry, and protected. Monitor for worsening condition.

NECROTIC TISSUE ON ISCHEMIC LIMBS

If ischemia is present, monitor wounds for signs and symptoms of worsening condition. If the wound is eschar-covered without signs of infection, keep the site clean, dry, and protected. If the wound is open, wound gel may be used. The wound will not heal without an adequate blood supply, but not all patients are candidates for surgery. Remember that aggressive wound care may, in fact, hasten the time of amputation.

WOUNDS/PRESSURE ULCERS ON PATIENTS AT THE END OF THEIR LIFE

Choose a dressing that is appropriate treatment for the wound, that will be comfortable for the patient, and that reduces the frequency of dressing changes. For a heavily exuding wound, a calcium alginate dressing would absorb drainage, keep the patient comfortable, and reduce the frequency of dressing changes. If the wound is dry, a gel would keep the wound moist, be comfortable, and protect the wound. A specialty mattress for pressure reduction or pressure relief could prevent further breakdown and be comfortable for the patient.

and fluffed for maximum absorption capacity. When applied as a wet- to-dry dressing, they can facilitate debridement. When applied as a wet-to-moist or damp dressing, they act as moisture-retentive dressings. Gauze is available (sterile, non-sterile, in bulk, and with or without an adhesive border).

Purpose

1. cleansing
2. packing
3. covering
4. debriding

Absorbency

Depending upon the design of the dressing, light to moderate.

Uses

1. Stage II–IV pressure ulcers
2. lower extremity ulcers
3. surgical wounds
4. infected wounds

Cautions

1. Do not use on skin tears.
2. Avoid using on most graft sites.

Examples

- Curity Cover Sponges (Kendall)
- Curity Gauze Sponges (Kendall)
- Carrington Bordered Gauze (Carrington Laboratories, Inc.)
- Kerlex (Kendall)
- Medline Gauze Sponges (Medline Industries, Inc.)

TIPS
- Use high-quality 100 percent cotton, tightly woven, 12-ply gauze.
- To pack wounds, gauze should be opened, fluffed, and loosely packed, obliterating dead space but allowing room for absorption and expansion. For deep wounds, only one long dressing piece should be used. If several small dressing pieces are used, one may be left behind when dressing changes are made, which can lead to infection in the wound.
- A wet-to-dry dressing is one in which the gauze is moistened, placed into tunnels or undermined areas or applied to the wound, and allowed to dry. The dressing is then removed dry, without moistening the dressing on removal (in wet, out dry) to debride necrotic tissue.

IMPREGNATED GAUZES

Purpose

Gauzes can be impregnated with a variety of substances including petroleum, sodium chloride, and antiseptics to achieve a variety of healing goals. Most impregnated gauzes are designed to promote a moist healing environment and to facilitate ease in dressing removal without disruption of healing tissue. (See Appendix 5–A, page 83.) They are nonadherent and require a secondary dressing.

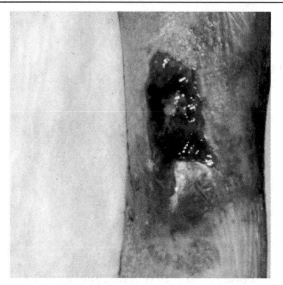

Figure 5–1 Skin Tear with Hypergranulation Tissue. Note fragile "onion peel" type skin surrounding the wound.

Clinical Objectives:
(1) Clean
(2) Protect wound and surrounding skin
(3) Manage exudate
(4) Manage hypergranulation tissue
See Color Plate 8.

Absorbency

1. moderate (most)
2. high (crystalline sodium chloride)

Uses

Refer to Table 5–1, page 56 to match kinds of impregnated gauzes to wound types. Impregnated gauzes can be used on the following kinds of wounds:

1. Stage II–IV pressure ulcers
2. lower extremity ulcers
3. surgical wounds
4. skin tears (moist products only)
5. grafts
6. infected wounds (particularly crystalline sodium chloride)

Caution

Crystalline sodium chloride is inappropriate for dry wounds.

Examples

- Absorb-A-Salt™ (Dumex Medical)
- ADAPTIC™ (Johnson & Johnson Medical)
- Xeroform Petrolatum Gauze (Kendall)
- Mesalt® (Mölnlycke)
- Vaseline Gauze Dressing (Kendall)
- Dermagran Hydraphillic Wound Dressing (Derma Sciences)

TIPS • Always follow manufacturer's recommendations for use and frequency of change.
- Nonadherent impregnated gauze may be refrigerated and may help to decrease pain at the wound site.

ALGINATES

Alginates are composed of natural polysaccharide fibers or are derived from seaweed. They are composed of soft, nonwoven fibers shaped as rope or pads. Alginates are highly absorbent and conform to the shape of the wound. When placed into a wound, an alginate generally interacts with wound exudate to form a gel that maintains a moist healing environment. There must be enough exudate in the wound to convert the dry alginate fibers into a gel. They can require a secondary dressing.

Purpose

1. packing (fills dead space)
2. absorption (absorbs up to 20 times its weight)
3. maintaining moist environment (forms a gel within the wound and facilitates autolytic debridement)

Absorbency

moderate to high

Uses

1. Stage II–IV pressure ulcers

2. lower extremity ulcers
3. surgical wounds
4. infected wounds
5. diabetic ulcers

Caution

A gel will not form in a dry wound.

Examples

- AlgiDERM® (Bard)
- Kaltostat® (ConvaTec)
- Sorbsan (Bertek)
- Hyperion® (Hyperion Medical)
- Restore CalciCare Calcium Alginate Dressing (Hollister, Inc.)
- Kalginate (DeRoyal)
- Carasorb (Kendall)
- Ferris PolyMem Calcium Alginate Dressing (Ferris Mfg. Corp.)

TIPS • Alginates are available in many configurations and sizes, making them practical for a multitude of wounds requiring packing.
- Alginates may be flushed from the wound with normal saline.
- They can often be useful to decrease the frequency of dressing changes—most can remain in the wound until drainage is seen on the outer dressing.
- They are useful under compression wraps.

ANTIMICROBIALS

Antimicrobials can come as creams, ointments, impregnated gauzes, or other types of dressings.

Purpose

1. to control/reduce the number of microorganisms in a wound without damaging healthy tissue
2. to maintain a moist healing environment

Absorbency

1. Depending upon the dressing, low to high
2. Can require a secondary dressing

Uses

1. Stage II–IV pressure ulcers
2. lower extremity ulcers
3. surgical wounds
4. skin tears
5. grafts
6. infected wounds

Cautions

1. Read the manufacturer's recommendations.
2. Precautions must be taken when using iodine-based antimicrobials if there is a risk that the patient has a thyroid disorder.
3. These products are not intended to treat systemic infection.

Examples

- Thermazene Cream ("Silvadene") (Kendall)
- Iodoflex™ (Healthpoint)
- Iodosorb® (Healthpoint)
- Arglaes (Medline Industries, Inc.)
- Acticoat 7 (Smith & Nephew, Inc.)
- Acticoat Absorbent Dressing (Smith & Nephew, Inc.)
- Actisorb (Johnson & Johnson Medical)
- Kerlex AMD (Kendall)
- SilvaSorb Antimicrobial Silver Dressing (Medline Industries, Inc.)
- Silverlon Wound Pad Dressing (Argentum Medical LLC)

FOAMS

Foam dressings are nonlinting and absorbent. Foams create a moist environment and provide thermal insulation to the wound. They are manufactured as pads, sheets, and pillow (cavity) dressings. They are generally nonadherent, may repel contaminants, are easy to apply and remove, absorb light to heavy amounts of exudate, and may be used under compression. They can be layered in combination with other materials. They also can have an adhesive border or a transparent film coating.

Purpose

1. absorb exudate
2. promote moist healing environment

Absorbency

high

Uses

1. Stage II–IV pressure ulcers
2. lower extremity ulcers
3. skin tears

Cautions

1. Do not use on dry wounds.
2. Do not use with infected wounds.
3. Do not use as packing unless the product is specifically designed and labeled for packing, such as pillow "cavity" dressings.

Examples

- Allevyn (Smith & Nephew, Inc.)
- PolyMem® (Ferris Mfg. Corp.)
- Cutinova® Foam (Beiersdorf-Jobst)
- Flexzan® (Bertek)
- Lyofoam® (ConvaTec)
- 3M Foam Dressing–Adhesive or Nonadhesive (3M Health Care)
- Biatain Foam Dressing (Coloplast)
- Curaforam Foam Dressing (Kandall)
- Tielle Hydropolymer Adhesive and Borderless Nonadhesive (Johnson & Johnson Medical)
- Mepilex–Borfer and Soft Silicone Absorbent Form Dressing (Mölnlycke Health Care)
- Polyderm–Plus and Border (DeRoyal)

TIPS	• Foams are easy to use and easy to teach patients/caregivers to use.
	• Most are nonadherent, and they are available in many sizes and configurations.
	• They are useful in decreasing the frequency of dressing changes, and most can be left in place until approximately 75 percent saturated.

HYDROCOLLOIDS

These are occlusive or semiocclusive dressings composed of materials such as gelatin, pectin, and/or carboxymethylcellulose. They generally provide a moist healing environment that allows clean wounds to granulate and necrotic wounds to debride autolytically. They are generally impermeable to bacteria and other contaminants. They are permeable to moisture vapor, but not water. Hydrocolloids may be left in place for three to five days and may be used under compression. Absorbency depends upon composition. These dressings are self adhering and available with and without a border. They contour easily.

Purpose

1. autolytic debridement
2. maintenance of moist healing environment
3. protection of the wound from external contaminants

Absorbency

1. low to moderate
2. may be enhanced with use of hydrocolloid paste

Uses

1. Stage I–III pressure ulcers
2. venous stasis ulcers

Cautions

1. Do not use on arterial or neuropathic ulcers.
2. Do not use if there is fragile skin surrounding the wound.
3. Do not use on infected wounds.

Examples

- DuoDERM® CGF® (ConvaTec)
- Restore™ (Hollister, Inc.)
- Comfeel® (Coloplast)
- OriDerm (Orion Medical Products)
- 3M Tegasorb™ (3M Health Care)
- Exuderm (Medline Industries, Inc.)
- NuDerm (Johnson & Johnson Medical)

TIPS
- Always use a larger size than the size of the wound; at least a 1-inch margin of hydrocolloid is needed. In difficult areas, up to a 3-inch margin may be needed for good adherence.
- You may need to create a picture frame with paper tape or transparent film.
- Many varieties are available in thin, conformable styles, often contoured to fit surface areas.
- Hydrocolloids may be useful under Montgomery straps to protect skin from adhesive.
- If used on "cratered" wounds, dead space must be filled in with hydrocolloid paste or alginate.

HYDROFIBERS

Hydrofibers are sterile nonwoven pads or ribbons composed of sodium carboxymethylcellulose fibers. They are conformable and absorbent and they interact with wound exudate to form a gel. There must be enough exudate in the wound to convert the hydrofiber into a gel.

Purpose

1. packing
2. absorption
3. maintenance of a moist environment
4. autolytic debridement

Absorbency

high

Uses

1. Stage II–IV pressure ulcers
2. lower extremity ulcers
3. surgical wounds

Cautions

1. Do not use on dry wounds.
2. Do not use on infected wounds.

Example

Aquacel™ Hydrofiber™ (ConvaTec)

TIPS • Select a size that is at least an inch larger than the wound.
• If packing, do so lightly, do not overfill, and do not apply with pressure.
• Hydrofibers may be left in place for several days depending on the amount of exudate. If it does not become a gel-like sheet, flush it out with saline and consider using a less absorbent product.

HYDROGELS

Hydrogels are polymers, water- or glycerin-based amorphous gels, impregnated gauzes, or sheet dressings. They do not absorb large amounts of exudate because of their high water content. They help maintain a moist wound environment and promote granulation and epithelialization. Most dressings are soothing, reduce pain, rehydrate the wound bed, fill in dead spaces (impregnated gauze), and are easy to apply and remove. They generally require a secondary dressing.

Purpose

1. autolytic debridement
2. maintenance of a moist healing environment
3. hydration of dry wounds

Absorbency

low

Uses

1. Stage II–IV pressure ulcers
2. lower extremity ulcers
3. skin tears (in particular, sheet-style hydrogels)
4. surgical wounds

Caution

Do not use on heavily exudating wounds.

Examples

*   Biolex™ (Bard)
*   Carrasyn® (Carrington Laboratories, Inc.)
*   Curasol® (Healthpoint)
*   IntraSite (Smith & Nephew, Inc.)
*   SoloSite® (Smith & Nephew, Inc.)
*   Vigilon® (Bard)
*   Restore Hydrogel Dressing (Hollister, Inc.)
*   RadiGel (Carrington Laboratories, Inc.)
*   Curafil Hydrogel Impregnated Gauze (Kendall)
*   Curafil Gel Wound Dressing (Kendall)

TIPS • Hydrogels are available in sheets, impregnated gauze, and amorphous gel. Select the most appropriate form for the type and location of the wound.
  • They may be refrigerated to enhance the soothing, pain-relieving property of the dressing.

TRANSPARENT FILMS

These adhesive, semipermeable, polyurethane membrane dressings vary in size and configuration. They are waterproof and are impermeable to contaminants and bacteria. However, they permit water vapor and atmospheric gases to cross the barrier. They do not absorb drainage. They retain moisture and are to be changed when fluid accumulates beneath them. Because these dressings are clear, wounds can be assessed without removing the dressing. They are available in a wide variety of sizes.

Purpose

1. encourages autolytic debridement
2. promotes moist healing environment
3. protects from external contaminants

Absorbency

low

Uses

1. Stage I–II pressure ulcers
2. partial-thickness wounds
3. skin tears (cautiously)
4. grafts
5. secondary, securing dressing over many other wound coverings

Cautions

1. Do not use on fragile skin surfaces.
2. Do not use on infected wounds.
3. Avoid using on wounds with large amounts of exudate.

Examples

- Tegaderm™ (3M Health Care)
- Bioclusive™ (Johnson & Johnson Medical)
- OpSite (Smith & Nephew, Inc.)
- DermaSite™ (Derma Sciences)
- Comfeel Film (Coloplast)
- Polyskin II Transparent Dressing (Kendall)
- BlisterFilm Transparent Dressing (Kendall)

TIPS
- It is normal for exudate to be present on the wound surface under a film dressing. If the drainage is on the intact skin surrounding the wound, the dressing should be changed.
- If excessive exudate is on the wound surface, a tuberculin syringe may be used to aspirate the drainage. The puncture site can then be patched.

ENZYMATIC DEBRIDERS

By digesting necrotic tissue, these ointments debride wounds. Different types of enzymatic agents include proteolytic enzymes, fibrinolytic enzymes, collagenase, and papain. Their actions are specific to necrotic tissue. Most manufacturers report that they do not damage healthy tissue. (See Appendix 5–B, page 85.)

Purpose

1. debridement of necrotic tissue without damaging healthy tissue
2. maintenance of moist healing environment

Absorbency

1. low
2. secondary dressing (usually gauze moistened with saline) always required

Use

- necrotic wounds
  - slough
  - eschar

Caution

Do not use on fully granular wounds. Enzymatic debriders will not harm granulation tissue, but they are no longer necessary when all necrotic tissue is removed.

Examples

- Collagenase Santyl® (Ross Products Division of Abbott Laboratories)
- Accuzyme® (Healthpoint)
- Panafil® (Healthpoint)

TIPS • Enzymatic debriders are available only by prescription, through a pharmacy.

- Be sure to follow the manufacturer's recommendations about the use of antimicrobials in conjunction with debriding agents.
- The enzymatic action of such agents may be affected by the presence of salts, heavy metals, and antimicrobials.
- Hard eschar should be scored or crosshatched to allow the enzymes to be effective.

GROWTH FACTORS

Growth factors are proteins that occur naturally in the human body. They cause cellular growth and cell migration and may regulate the wound healing process. They can be obtained through a process utilizing the body's platelets and macrophages, atologously derived, or made chemically or biochemically outside of the body, recombinant. Use of a growth factor is an adjunct to standard wound practice, such as debridement, pain relief, and infection control.

Purpose

1. cell proliferation
2. acceleration of healing

Absorbency

1. low
2. covered with moist gauze dressing

Use

clean, granulating wounds only

Cautions

1. Do not use on necrotic wounds.
2. Do not use on cancer sites, or with patients with any neoplasms.
3. Store at reduced temperatures.

Example

Regranex® (Ortho-McNeil Pharmaceutical) (See Exhibit 5–2, page 74.)

TIPS	• Growth factors are not effective on necrotic tissue.
	• They are available by prescription only.
	• Close adherence to manufacturer's instructions is imperative.

BIOSYNTHETICS

These may be gels or semiocclusive sheets derived from a natural source and may require freezing. They are used primarily on burn wounds and have also been found effective on a variety of skin-loss wounds, including skin tears and donor sites. They act as a skin substitute. They foster healing by re-epithelialization. They may be nonadherent. The product is surgically applied to the wound surface by a physician and covered with a dressing.

Examples

- Biobrane® (Bertek)
- BGC Matrix® (Brennen Medical Inc.)
- Inerpan® (Kendall)
- Apligraf® (Novartis)

COLLAGEN

Collagen is a fibrous, insoluble protein produced by fibroblasts and is derived from bovine hide. Collagen dressings may stimulate new tissue development and wound debridement. Collagen dressings may encourage the deposition and organization of newly formed collagen fibers and granulation tissue in the wound bed. The dressings absorb exudate and maintain a moist wound-healing environment. The dressing can be 100 percent collagen or combined with other products such as alginates. They are nonadherent and are easy to apply and remove. Examples include

Examples

- Fibracol™ (Johnson & Johnson Medical)
- Cellerete Rx (Hymed Group Corp.)
- Promogran Matrix Wound Dressing (Johnson & Johnson Medical)

Caution

Do not use on dry wounds or with patients sensitive to bovine products.

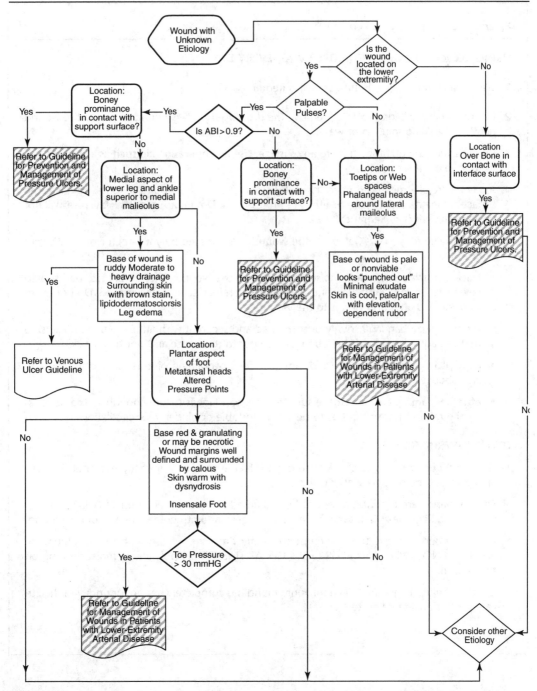

Figure 5–2 Local Wound Managment Interventions Algorithm. (Courtesy of Bonnie Sue Ralstad, RN, BA, CWOCN Copyright © 2000)

Exhibit 5–2 Patient Guide: Regranex®

USING REGRANEX® GEL THE PROPER WAY, EVERY DAY

1. Wash hands thoroughly before applying Regranex® Gel.

2. Before you apply Regranex® Gel, remove the dressing from the wound and rinse the wound gently with saline solution or water.

3. Do not touch the tip of the tube to any surface. Use an application aid such as a cotton swab or tongue depressor.

4. Apply a carefully measured quantity of Regranex® Gel to the wound (enough to cover the surface) as instructed by your health care professional. Do not apply a thick layer—it will not increase the effect of Regranex® Gel.

5. After applying Regranex® Gel, dress the wound as instructed by your doctor or health care professional.

   - Place a suitable size, saline-moistened pad over the wound. The correct size pad should cover the wound completely and have at least an inch to spare all around. Do not try to trim the pad after applying it to the wound.

   - Wrap a gauze bandage snugly over the pad and secure it with adhesive tape. Make sure that the adhesive side of the tape is secured onto the gauze and not to your skin.

   - Only plain gauze should be used. Any dressings containing ointments or other ingredients should be avoided.

   - After bandaging, check to make sure that the bandage is secure enough so that it doesn't slip off, but not so tight as to be uncomfortable or hinder your circulation.

OTHER INSTRUCTIONS

- You should use a mirror to check both of your feet every day. Adjust the mirror at different angles to get the best view of your feet.

- Other wound care products have not been studied for use with Regranex® Gel. Therefore, when using Regranex® Gel, avoid other creams, gels, or ointments at the site of the wound.

- After 12 hours, remove the dressing and gently rinse the wound with saline solution or water. DO NOT APPLY ANY REGRANEX® GEL AT THIS TIME. Apply a new moist dressing on the wound.

- Continue to use Regranex® Gel until your wound has completely healed, or until your health care professional tells you to stop.

continues

Exhibit 5–2 continued

- Visit your health care professional regularly during the course of treatment.

- If you feel any discomfort, or have any questions, contact your health care professional immediately.

- Regranex® Gel must be stored in the refrigerator at all times. DO NOT FREEZE.

QUESTIONS & ANSWERS

Q. **What is Regranex® Gel, and what does it do for diabetic foot ulcers?**

A. Regranex® Gel is a prescription drug for the treatment of diabetic foot ulcers. It contains a factor normally found in the blood (referred to as a platelet-derived growth factor), which is part of the body's natural healing process. Some wounds take a long time to heal and others may not heal at all. Regranex® Gel can help this problem in many patients by delivering the growth factor directly to the ulcer in a simple-to-use gel.

Q. **How is Regranex® Gel different from other wound care therapies?**

A. You may have heard of, or even tried, other treatments for diabetic foot ulcers. Most of these treatments only help keep the wound clean and moist. Regranex® Gel is different because it is clinically proven to help heal more wounds.

Q. **What, if any, side effects can I expect from using Regranex® Gel?**

A. When used correctly, Regranex® Gel is well tolerated. A small percentage of patients treated with Regranex® Gel experienced local irritation or rash. If you experience any such effect, you should discuss it with your doctor or health care professional.

RELATED WOUND TREATMENTS

Vacuum-Controlled Assisted Closure—V.A.C.

V.A.C. therapy is a system that uses controlled negative pressure (vacuum) to help promote wound healing. This system consists of a computer-controlled therapy unit, canister, sterile plastic tubing, foam dressing, and clear V.A.C. drape. The foam dressing goes inside the wound. One end of the tube connects to the foam. The other end of the tube connects to the canister, which in turn, connects to the V.A.C. system. The wound area is sealed with clear V.A.C. drape similar to a large bandage. The V.A.C. system then pulls infectious materials and excess interstitial fluid from the wound through the tube and collects them inside the canister.

Clinical benefits of V.A.C. therapy can include:

- Decreased edema of periwound area
- Increased local vascularity
- Decreased bacterial colonization
- Increased rate of granulation tissue formation
- Maintenance of moist wound environment
- Increased rate of contraction
- Accurate measurement of wound drainage

Indications

- Dehisced surgical wounds
- Complex operative wounds left open to heal by secondary intention
- Diabetic ulcers
- Chronic wounds
- Acute wounds
- Pressure ulcers
- Flaps and grafts
- Chronic or acute enteric fistulas

Contraindications

- Malignancy
- Untreated osteomyelitis
- Fistulas to organs or body cavities
- Necrotic tissue with eschar present
- Exposed arteries or veins
- Uncontrolled pain

Precautions should be taken with patients exhibiting:

- Active bleeding
- Difficult hemostasis
- Anticoagulant therapy

When placing the V.A.C. dressing in proximity to blood vessels, the clinician should take care to ensure that all vessels are adequately protected with overlying fascia, tissue, or other protective barriers. Greater care should be taken with respect to weakened, irradiated, or sutured blood vessels. Follow universal precautions.

Tips

Wound site should be inspected for signs of infection with each dressing change. Any changes should be reported to physician. Typically the V.A.C. dressing is changed every 24 to 72 hours, with the exception of infected wounds. Infected wounds are changed every 12 to 24 hours. If the V.A.C. dressing adheres to the wound, try wetting the dressing with normal saline, or use nonadherent porous material between the dressing and the wound. Always replace the dressings with V.A.C. sterile disposables from unopened packages. Teach the patient and/or caregiver how to check the dressing to maintain an adequate seal. Keep therapy on. Never leave off for more than two hours per day. Remove the V.A.C. dressing if unable to maintain a vacuum, or if therapy is off for more than two hours. To optimize healing outcomes with the V.A.C., refer to the chapter on basic wound care, especially as it relates to nutrition, wound cleansing, and pressure relief.

The patient can have V.A.C. therapy started at the hospital, extended care, or home. If started at the hospital, the V.A.C. therapy can be transitioned home or to an extended care facility.

Wound V.A.C. therapy is specialized wound care. Follow all applicable manuals and reference guides as to product use and application. Be sure to consult the patient's treating physician as to individual conditions and treatment.

For further information see the bibliography at the end of this chapter. KCI website: www.woundvac.com. Contact: 1-877-WOUNDVAC or 1-877-968-6382 for 24-hour, 7-day-a-week service for emergencies (such as equipment failure).

Noncontact Normothermic Wound Therapy (NNWT)

NNWT is a wound management system that uses a special heated bandage to provide controlled, radiant warmth to a wound within an optimal moist environment of 100 percent humidity. The moist environment can facilitate autolytic debridement. The heating element uses an infrared heater to warm the wound to one degree above normal. Warming encourages blood vessels to dilate, increasing blood flow and oxygen to the periwound area.

Indications

NNWT is indicated for full and partial-thickness wounds including Stage II-IV pressure ulcers; venous, arterial, and neuropathic/diabetic ulcers; and surgical wounds. It may be used on clinically infected wounds with concurrent-appropriate antibiotic therapy.

Contraindications

NNWT is not indicated for use in third-degree burns or stable arterial wounds with dry eschar.

The only commercially available product to deliver NNWT is Warm-Up therapy (Augustine Medical, Eden Prairie, MN).

Hyperbaric Oxygen (HBO)

Hyperbaric oxygen therapy is inhalation of 100% oxygen delivered at pressures of more than 1 atmosphere (ATA). Hyperbaric oxygen is provided in enclosed chambers in individual (monoplace) and group (multiplace) settings. It is believed to promote wound healing by stimulating fibroblast, collagen synthesis, epithelialization, and controlling infection.

Indications

HBO has been around for a long time, but it remains controversial because of a limited evidence base. Despite this, the American Diabetic Association indicated that adjunctive HBO may be reasonable to use in treating severe limb- or life-threatening wounds that haven't responded to other treatments. Other wounds that respond to HBO are those that have been acutely or chronically compromised by hypoxia and/or infection. Clinical conditions associated with these types of wounds are peripheral vascular disease, diabetes, radiation necrosis, mixed soft tissue infections, refractory osteomyelitis, and selected traumatic wounds.

The costs of a nonhealing wound are great. HBO may be considered in combination with good wound care when traditional wound treatment plans have failed.

COMPOSITES

A composite is a combination of two or more physically distinct products manufactured as a single dressing that provides multiple functions.

Examples

- Covaderm Plus® (DeRoyal Wound Care)
- Alldress® Absorbent Film Dressing (Mölnlycke)
- Visasorb Wound Dressing (Kendall)
- CovRSite Plus Composite Dressing (Smith & Nephew, Inc.)
- Repel Wound Dressing (MPM Medical Sciences, Inc.)

COMPRESSION WRAPS

Compression wraps help to heal venous ulcers by reducing dependent edema and facilitating venous return through the enhancement of the effects of the foot and calf muscle pumps. They are available as single or multiple layers and elastic stockings. More information is found in Chapter 8, Exhibit 8–1, page 159.

Examples

- Profore Four Layer Bandaging System (Smith & Nephew, Inc.)
- Unna-flex® Elastic Unna Boot (ConvaTec)
- CircAid® (Coloplast)
- Jobst® UlcerCare (Beiersdorf-Jobst, Inc.)
- Dyna-flex™ Multi-Layer Compression System (Johnson & Johnson Medical)

Caution

Contraindicated with arterial disease.

Exhibit 5–3 Teaching Guide for Topical Treatments*

	Instructions Given (Date/Initials)	Demonstration or Review of Materials (Date/Initials)	Return Demonstration or States Understanding (Date/Initials)

1. Type of Wound
2. Types of Wound Dressings
  a. Alginate
  b. Films
  c. Foams
  d. Gauze
  e. Hydrogel
  f. Hydrocolloid
3. Reason for Dressing
  a. Maintain dryness
  b. Add moisture
  c. Retain moisture
  d. Absorb moisture			

Exhibit 5–3 continued

	Instructions Given (Date/Initials)	Demonstration or Review of Materials (Date/Initials)	Return Demonstration or States Understanding (Date/Initials)

4. Wound Care
  a. Demonstrates ability to cleanse a wound
  b. Demonstrates ability to apply a wound dressing and topical agents
  c. Demonstrates ability to protect surrounding skin from maceration
  d. Demonstrates ability to make and record simple wound measurements			

5. Infection Prevention
  a. Demonstrates proper handwashing before and after handling soiled dressings
  b. Understands universal precautions
  c. Knows how to dispose of infectious waste
  d. Recognizes/describes warning signs of local infection: pain, swelling, pus, and warmth
  e. Recognizes signs of systemic infection: lethargy, confusion, elevated temperature
  f. Understands when to call the health care professional if infection is suspected			

6. Wound Drainage and Tissue Types a. Recognizes and reports accurately the amount of wound drainage			

Exhibit 5–3 continued

	Instructions Given (Date/Initials)	Demonstration or Review of Materials (Date/Initials)	Return Demonstration or States Understanding (Date/Initials)
b. Recognizes tissue types and goals: black (dry) = dead → soften, clean yellow/tan (soft) = dead → clean red/pink (moist) = healthy → protect			
7. Universal Precautions a. Handwashing b. Use of gloves and protective equipment during care procedures c. Disposal of contaminated materials			
8. Wound Cleansing a. Shallow wound: cleanse gently from center to edge with saline b. Deep wound: uses syringe to flush and then gently massages out extra fluids			
9. When to Notify the Health Care Provider a. Signs and symptoms of infection b. Failure to improve c. Presence of odor d. Pus (drainage) e. Large amount of pus (drainage) f. Elevated temperature or signs of confusion in the older adult			
10. Will Make Appointment to Return for Follow-up Care			

*Must be individualized for each patient and caregiver.

REFERENCES

Bergstrom, N. et al. 1994. *Treatment of pressure ulcers.* Clinical Practice Guideline No. 15. AHCPR Publication No. 95-0652. Rockville, MD: U.S. Department of Health and Human Services. Public Health Services, Agency for Health Care Policy and Research.

Boykin, J. V. 2001. Treatment options and questions and answers about hyperbaric oxygen therapy. *Advances in Skin and Wound Care.* 14(5), 232–234.

Mendez-Eastman, S. 2001. Guidelines for using negative pressure wound therapy. *Advances in Skin and Wound Care.* 14(6), 314–325.

Whitney, J. D. et al. 2001. Pressure ulcers with noncontact normothermic wound therapy: Healing and warming effects. *Journal of WOCN Wound, Ostomy & Continence Nursing* 28(5), 244–252.

BIBLIOGRAPHY

Baranoski, S. 1999. Wound dressings: Challenging decisions. *Home Healthcare Nurse* 17, no. 1: 19–25.

Baranoski, S., & Ayello, E. A. 2004. Wound treatment options. In S. Baranoski & E. A. Ayello (Eds.) *Wound care essentials: Practice principles* (127–156) Philadelphia: Lippincott Williams & Wilkens.

Hess, C. 1997. *Wound care: Nurse's clinical guide,* 2d ed. Springhouse, PA: Springhouse Corp.

Houghton, P., and K. Campbell. 1999. Choosing an adjunctive therapy for the treatment of chronic wounds. *Ostomy/Wound Management* 45, no. 8: 43–52.

Rolstad, B. S., Ovington, L. G., & Harris, A. 2000. Wound care product formulary. In R. A. Bryant (Ed.) *Acute and chronic wounds: Nursing management* (2nd ed.) (113–124). St. Louis, MO: Mosby, Inc.

Sibbald, R. 1998. An approach to leg and foot ulcers: A brief overview. *Ostomy/Wound Management* 44, no. 9: 28–35.

Sprung, P. et al. 1998. Hydrogels and hydrocolloids: An objective products comparison. *Ostomy/Wound Management* 44, no. 1: 36–53.

Sussman, C., and B. Bates-Jensen. 1998. *Wound care: A collaborative practice manual for physical therapists and nurses.* Gaithersburg, MD: Aspen Publishers, Inc.

Van Rijswijk, L., and J. Beitz. 1998. The traditions and terminology of wound dressings: Food for thought. *Journal of Wound Ostomy and Continence Nursing* 25: 116–122.

Resources/Manufacturer's List

Manufacturer	Phone	Website
3M Health Care	1-800-228-3957	www.3M.com/healthcare
Bard Medical Division	1-800-526-4455	www.bardmedical.com
B. Braun/McGaw	1-800-227-2862	www.bbraunsa.com
Beiersdorf-Jobst, Inc.	1-800-537-1063	www.beiersdorf.com
Bertek Pharmaceuticals	1-888-823-7835	www.bertek.com
Brennen Medical Inc.	1-800-328-9105	www.brennenmedical.com
BioCore Medical Technologies, Inc.	1-888-565-5243	www.biocore.com
Carrington Labs	1-800-527-5216	www.carringtonlabs.com
Coloplast	1-800-533-0464	www.coloplast.com
ConvaTec	1-800-422-8811	www.convatec.com
Derma Sciences, Inc.	1-800-825-4325	www.dermasciences.com
DeRoyal Wound Care	1-800-337-6925	www.deroyal.com
Dumex Medical	1-800-463-0106	www.dumex.com
Ferris Manufacturing Corp.	1-800-765-9636	www.ferriscares.com
Healthpoint	1-800-441-8227	www.healthpoint.com
Hollister, Inc.	1-800-323-4060	www.hollister.com
Hymed Group Corp.	1-610-865-9876	www.hymed.com
Hyperion Medical Inc.	1-800-743-8111	www.hyperionmedical.com
Johnson & Johnson Medical Division of Ethicon, Inc.	1-800-255-2500	www.jnjwoundcare.com
Kendall Health Care Products, Inc.	1-800-962-9888	www.kendallhq.com
Knoll Pharmaceuticals	1-800-372-6895	www.knoll-pharma.com
Medline Industries, Inc.	1-800-633-5463	www.medline.net
Mölnlycke	1-800-992-9939	www.molnlyckehc.com
Novartis	1-888-432-5232	www.apligraf.com
Orion Medical Products	1-800-669-5079	www.orimed.com
Ortho-McNeil Pharmaceutical Inc.	1-888-734-7263	www.regranex.com
Smith & Nephew, Inc.	1-800-876-1261	www.snwmd.com

Patient Guide: Santyl®, Accuzyme®, Panafil®, and Iodoflex Gel and Iodosorb Pads

SANTYL®

Caring for the Skin Ulcer

These instructions are general; be sure to follow your health care professional's directions for your specific condition.

Change the dressing on the skin ulcer at least once every day. If the area becomes soiled or damp, change the dressing as often as needed, and follow all of the steps below.

A health care professional may need to cut through some of the dead tissue in the skin ulcer and remove as much of it as possible. This should not be painful. DO NOT try to do this yourself.

1. Wash your hands with soap and water. Dry with a clean towel.

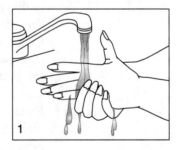

2. Gently clean the open wound according to instructions specified by your health care professional.

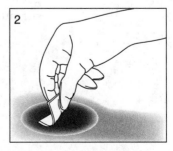

3. Rinse the wound with normal saline solution (your health care professional can tell you how to obtain or make this) to remove any dead skin.

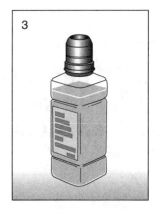

4. If you have been instructed to use an antibiotic powder on the area, sprinkle a light dusting of powder onto the wound area.

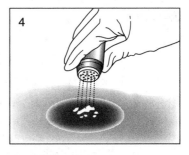

5. Apply Santyl® ointment:
   a. *For a shallow wound,* put Santyl® ointment on a sterile gauze pad, and then apply it directly to the wound, so that the ointment touches the ulcer surface. Do not get the ointment on the surrounding skin.
   b. *For a deep ulcer,* use a clean wooden tongue depressor to gently apply Santyl® ointment to the wound surface. Do not get the ointment on the surrounding skin. Throw

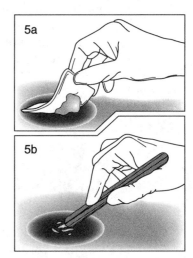

the tongue depressor away
with the soiled dressing in a
closed plastic bag.

6. Cover the wound with a
dry, sterile gauze pad.
Secure the pad with nonal-
lergenic paper tape. Use as
little tape as possible
to keep the dressing in
place. Leave the sides of
the gauze pad open.

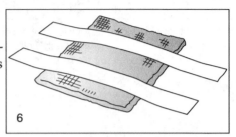

Is Your Ulcer Getting Better?

A skin ulcer can be like an iceberg: There may be a large area below
the surface of the ulcer that is not easily seen. In order for healing to take
place below the surface, the dead skin on the top has to be removed first.
That's part of the job of Santyl® ointment—to clear away the dead tissue
cells.

When Santyl® ointment is used properly, the wound might get bigger
at first. This is actually a good sign. So is an unpleasant odor—it means
the wound is draining and getting cleaner, and that's a positive step in the
healing process.

As the dead tissue disappears, healthy pink skin cells will start to
form around the edges of the wound. With time and proper care, healthy
tissue will fill in the wound.

The Healing Process Over Time

1. The skin ulcer is filled with dead skin.
2. Antibiotic fights infection and Santyl® ointment removes dead
    skin.
3. Healthy pink cells start to form around the edge and on the sur-
    face. Santyl® ointment can be used, as per the package insert
    (PDR), until granulation tissue is well established.
4. Healthy skin tissue fills in the wound.

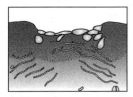

1. The skin ulcer is filled with dead skin.

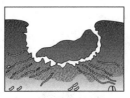

2. Antibiotic fights infection and Santyl® ointment removes dead skin.

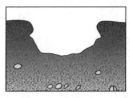

3. Healthy pink cells start to form around the edge and on the surface. Discontinue Santyl® when granulation tissue is well established.

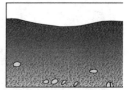

4. Healthy skin tissue fills in the wound.

ACCUZYME®

Accuzyme® Papain-Urea and Debriding Ointment is suggested topical treatment in acute and chronic wounds such as pressure ulcers, burns, postoperative wounds, varicose and diabetic ulcers, and miscellaneous traumatic and infected wounds. Accuzyme® is used for enzymatic debridement of necrotic (dead) tissue and slough.

Dosage and Administration

- Remove the old wound dressing carefully so as not to injure the wound or surrounding tissues.
- At each redressing, flush the wound with a lukewarm (not hot) saline (saltwater) solution or a mild cleansing solution to remove any accumulation of liquified dead tissue.
- Pat the area dry with clean gauze or a clean towel.
- Apply a thin layer of Accuzyme® ointment directly to the wound surface and cover with the appropriate dressing. Take care not to make the dressing too tight.
- Application once or twice daily is preferred.

Caution

Avoid use of Accuzyme® ointment with hydrogen peroxide solution.

Precautions

There are no known reasons not to use this product. In general, Accuzyme® ointment is well tolerated by most people. A small percentage of patients have experienced a temporary "burning" sensation. Occasionally the profuse drainage produced by the digestion and liquification of the dead tissue may cause irritation to the surrounding skin. In such cases, more frequent dressing changes should be performed until the drainage diminishes. This will usually relieve the discomfort.

Note: Health care professionals may want to crosshatch (cut) into dead tissue before start of treatment.

If you have any questions about your wound or your reaction to this treatment, call your health care professional.

How Supplied

Accuzyme® ointment is available by prescription only.

PANAFIL®

Panafil® Debriding, Deodorizing, and Healing Ointment is suggested topical treatment for acute and chronic wounds such as varicose, diabetic, and pressure ulcers; burns; postoperative wounds; and miscellaneous traumatic and infected wounds. Panafil® Ointment is used to keep the wound clean of nonviable tissue and to promote normal healing.

Dosage and Administration

- Remove the old wound dressing carefully so as not to injure the wound or surrounding tissues.
- At each redressing, the wound should be flushed with a lukewarm (not hot) saline (saltwater) solution or a mild cleansing solution to remove any accumulation of liquified dead tissue.
- Pat the area dry with clean gauze or a clean towel.
- Apply a thin layer (⅛ inch of Panafil® Ointment) directly to the wound surface and cover with the appropriate dressing. Take care not to make the dressing too tight.

- Application once or twice daily is preferred, but longer intervals between dressing changes and reapplication have proved
  satisfactory.

Precautions

There are no known reasons not to use this product. In general,
Panafil® Ointment is well tolerated by most people. A small percentage of
patients have experienced a temporary "burning" sensation. Occasionally
the profuse drainage produced by the digestion and liquification of the
dead tissue may cause irritation to the surrounding skin. In such cases,
more frequent dressing changes should be performed until the drainage
diminishes. This will usually relieve the discomfort.

How Supplied

Panafil® ointment is available by prescription only.

IODOSORB Gel

Cadexomer Iodine

IODOFLEX Pads

Cadexomer Iodine

Iodosorb Gel and Iodoflex Pads are indicated for use in cleaning wet
ulcers and wounds such as venous stasis ulcers, pressure ulcers, diabetic
foot ulcers, infected traumatic wounds, and infected surgical wounds.
They cleanse draining and/or infected wounds by absorbing exudate
while actively fighting infection. They reduce the bacterial load through a
slow release of small amounts of a 0.9 percent elemental iodine into the
wound fluid. The patented, highly absorbent dressing has antimicrobial
action against staphylococcus aureus, streptococcus, pseudomonas
aeruginosa, and M.R.S.A.

Dosage and Administration

- Remove the old wound dressing carefully to prevent injury to the
  wound or the surrounding tissue. If necessary, soak the gauze for
  a few minutes; then remove.

- At each redressing, cleanse the wound with lukewarm saline solution or mild cleansing solution to remove debris from the wound bed.
- Pat the area dry with clean gauze.
- Apply Iodosorb Gel to at least ⅛-inch thickness over entire wound bed. Only ⅛ is required to achieve the desired effect, or if using Iodoflex Pad, remove the carrier gauze on one or both sides of the pad, and place the gel pad in contact with the wound surface. Any remaining Iodoflex should be discarded.
- Cover the wound with dry gauze or dressing of choice, and apply compression bandaging where appropriate.
- Change the dressing three times a week, or when all the Iodoflex/Iodosorb has changed in color from brown to yellow/gray. The number of applications should be reduced as the exudate diminishes.

Caution

Iodosorb Gel and Iodoflex Pads contain 0.9 percent weight-per-weight iodine, and should not be used on patients with known or suspected iodine sensitivity. Iodoflex is contraindicated in Hashimoto's thyroiditis, patients with a history of Graves Disease, or nontoxic nodular goiter. Patients with a history of any thyroid disorder are more susceptible to alteration in thyroid metabolism with chronic cadexomer iodine therapy. Neither Iodosorb or Iodoflex should be used in pregnant or lactating women because iodine is absorbed systemically.

Tips

- Wounds may appear larger during the first few days of treatment due to the reduction of edema.
- Neither Iodosorb or Iodoflex is effective in cleaning dry wounds.
- A small percentage of patients experience a slight transient pain during the first hour after application. In a few cases, moderate pain persisting for several hours has been reported.
- Always read the manufacturer's instructions prior to application the first time.

How Supplied

Iodosorb Gel and Iodoflex Pads are available by prescription only.

PART III

Wound Types Commonly Seen by Health Care Professionals

CHAPTER 6

Pressure Ulcers

Donna Oddo

Pressure ulcers, also commonly called decubitus ulcers, are areas where pressure has destroyed soft tissue. Typically located over bony prominences, pressure ulcers may occur in any area where pressure can adversely affect the soft tissue.

Assess all patients for their risk of skin breakdown upon admission and periodically throughout their length of care. Once a pressure ulcer develops, the patient is subject to increased pain and possible infection. This can lead to loss of function or loss of the limb, as well as fluid imbalances, malnourishment, and disfigurement. Patients may then require long-term nursing intervention and/or surgical intervention.

Prevention is imperative. Prevention measures should focus on reducing the pressure, maintaining and improving the patient's tissue tolerance to pressure, and educating the patient and caregiver.

ETIOLOGY

In normal tissue, a balance exists between interstitial and solid tissue pressure. Outside pressure forces can lead to

- an increase in interstitial fluid pressure
- a rise in arteriolar and capillary pressure
- filtering of a fluid from capillaries, resulting in
  - edema
  - autolysis
  - occlusion of lymph vessels
  - accumulation of anaerobic waste
  - necrosis

Approximately 70 percent of the tissue damage occurs below the skin surface.

ASSESSMENT

When staging a pressure ulcer (Exhibit 6–1, this page), remember:

- Stage the wound according to the depth of tissue damage visible.
- If damaged tissue is not visible, the wound cannot be staged. Necrotic tissue must be removed before damage can be assessed). (Figure 6–1; Color Plate 9.)
- It is inappropriate to backstage an ulcer as it heals. Stage is consistently kept at deepest level of damage: e.g., Stage IV will always be a Stage IV. The wound may fill with granulation tissue and close but will never be considered a Stage I, II, or III at any point in the healing process.

Exhibit 6–1 The Staging of Pressure Ulcers

These definitions of pressure ulcer stages are taken directly from the National Pressure Ulcer Advisory Panel. They are consistent with definitions used by the Agency for Health Care Policy and Research as well as the Wound Ostomy and Continence Nurse Society.

Stage I: An observable pressure-related alteration of intact skin whose indicators as compared to an adjacent or opposite area on the body may include changes in one or more of the following: skin temperature (warmth or coldness), tissue consistency (firm or boggy feel), and/or sensation (pain, itching). The ulcer appears as a defined area of persistent redness in lightly pigmented skin, whereas in darker skin tones, the ulcer may appear with persistent red, blue, or purple hues. (Figure 6–2; Color Plate 10.)

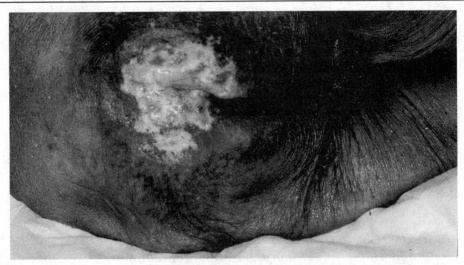

Figure 6–1 Pressure Ulcer on Sacrum. Necrotic center consistent with deeper tissue damage.
Clinical Objectives:
(1) Clean
(2) Remove slough
(3) Manage exudate
(4) Keep moist
(5) Protect from incontinence
(6) Relieve pressure
See Color Plate 9.

Exhibit 6–1 continued

Stage II: Partial-thickness skin loss involving epidermis, dermis, or both. The ulcer is superficial and presents clinically as an abrasion, lesion, or shallow crater (see Figure 6–3; Color Plate 11).

Stage III: Full-thickness skin loss involving damage to or necrosis of subcutaneous tissue that may extend down to, but not through, underlying fascia. The ulcer presents clinically as a deep crater with or without undermining the adjacent tissue. (Figure 6–4; Color Plate 12).

Stage IV: Full-thickness skin loss with extensive destruction, tissue necrosis, or damage to muscle, bone, or supporting structures (e.g., tendon, joint capsule). Undermining and sinus tracts also may be associated with Stage IV pressure ulcers. (Figure 6–5; Color Plate 13.)

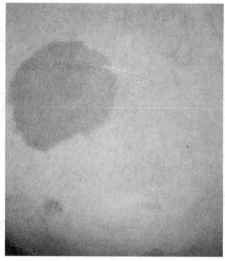

Figure 6–2 Stage I Pressure Ulcer. Nonblanchable erythema.

Clinical Objectives:

(1) Keep clean

(2) Cover and protect

(3) Eliminate pressure and friction

See Color Plate 10.

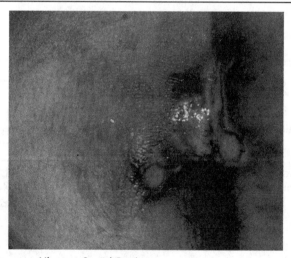

Figure 6–3 Stage II Pressure Ulcer at Sacral Region.

Clinical Objectives:

(1) Clean

(2) Protect from incontinence

(3) Keep moist

(4) Prevent pressure, friction, and shear.

See Color Plate 11.

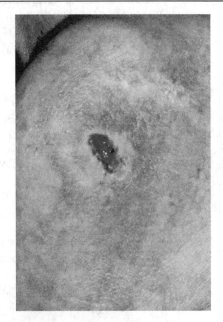

Figure 6–4 Healing Stage III Pressure Ulcer.
Clinical Objectives:
(1) Cleanse
(2) Keep moist
(3) Manage exudate
(4) Relieve pressure
See Color Plate 12.

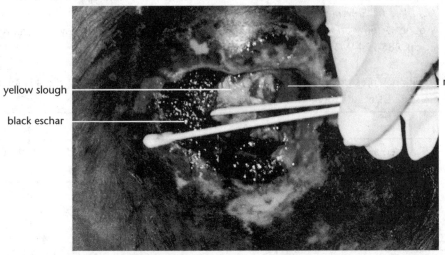

yellow slough

black eschar

red granulation tissue

Figure 6–5 Stage IV Pressure Ulcer on Sacrum with Necrotic Tissue and Undermining.
Clinical Objectives:
(1) Remove eschar
(2) Clean
(3) Keep moist
(4) Manage exudate
(5) Protect from incontinence
(6) Relieve pressure
See Color Plate 13.

BRADEN SCALE: HELPFUL TIPS When scoring each risk factor, if the assessment lies between two scores, use the lower score. When testing the patient's sensory perception, be sure to pinch the upper arm or thigh. Do not pinch fingers, hands, or nail beds. When testing the patient's sensory perception:

- if reflex response only, score 1
- if responds, but doesn't open eyes, score 3
- no paralysis, score 4

When testing the patient's activity:

- walks to bathroom or chair only, score 3

When testing mobility, do not consider the caregiver turning the patient.

- severe depression or medicated, score 2
- strongly prefers a position, score 3

When testing the patient's nutrition:

- usual intake—not temporary intake, e.g.; NPO for test

An excellent resource for prevention and treatment of pressure ulcers can be found in *Guideline for Prevention and Management of Pressure Ulcers.* Copyright 2002 by the Wound Ostomy and Continence Nurses Society. Refer to its website www.wocn.org, or call 888-224-WOCN.

Additional pressure ulcer assessment information can be found at the National Pressure Ulcer Advisory Panel web site, www.npuap.org.

TIP When a wound is obscured by necrotic tissue or is purple and indurated, document it as "unable to stage, consistent with deeper tissue damage."

PREVENTION

Assessing Risk

To identify at-risk patients, use one scale consistently, such as the Braden Scale (Exhibit 6–2, page 102),

- on admission

- on recertification or reactivation to services
- when the condition of the patient changes

To complete the Braden Scale:

1. In the last column, write the number that most closely matches the patient's condition.
2. Total the column.

   A total score of 16 or less is considered "at risk" (15 or 16 is considered low risk; 13 or 14 is considered moderate risk; and 12 or less is considered high risk).

TIP In home care, the scales broadly identify patients at risk. Be certain to assess factors in the home environment (e.g., caregiver ability and willingness, quality and amounts of oral intake, upkeep of patient's bedding and surroundings).

Risk Factors

Extrinsic Risk Factors

- pressure
- immobility
- limited mobility
- moisture
- heat
- friction
- shear

Intrinsic Risk Factors

- poor nutritional status (refer to the Nutritional Risk Screening Form [Exhibit 6–3, page 105])
- sensory deficit
- cardiopulmonary compromise
- anemia
- tissue fragility

TIP A good indicator of a patient's nutritional status is a serum pre-albumin or albumin level.

Exhibit 6–2 Braden Scale for Predicting Pressure Sore Risk

Patient's Name _____   Evaluator's Name _____   Date of Assessment _____

	1	2	3	4
SENSORY PERCEPTION ability to respond meaningfully to pressure-related discomfort	**1. Completely Limited:** Unresponsive (does not moan, flinch, or gasp) to painful stimuli, due to diminished level of consciousness or sedation. OR Limited ability to feel pain over most of body surface.	**2. Very Limited:** Responds only to painful stimuli. Cannot communicate discomfort except by moaning or restlessness. OR Has a sensory impairment that limits the ability to feel pain or discomfort over half the body.	**3. Slightly Limited:** Responds to verbal commands, but cannot always communicate discomfort or need to be turned. OR Has some sensory impairment that limits its ability to feel pain or discomfort in one or two extremities.	**4. No Impairment:** Responds to verbal commands. Has no sensory deficit that would limit ability to feel or voice pain or discomfort.
MOISTURE degree to which skin is exposed to moisture	**1. Constantly Moist:** Skin is kept moist almost constantly by perspiration, urine, etc. Dampness is detected every time patient is moved or turned.	**2. Very Moist:** Skin is often, but not always, moist. Linen must be changed at least once a shift.	**3. Occasionally Moist:** Skin is occasionally moist, requiring an extra linen change approximately once a day.	**4. Rarely Moist:** Skin is usually dry, linen only requires changing at routine intervals.

ACTIVITY degree of physical activity	**1. Bedfast:** Confined to bed.	**2. Chairfast:** Ability to walk severely limited or nonexistent. Cannot bear own weight and/or must be assisted into chair or wheelchair.	**3. Walks Occasionally:** Walks occasionally during day, but for very short distances, with or without assistance. Spends majority of each shift in bed or chair.	**4. Walks Frequently:** Walks outside the room at least twice a day and inside room at least every 2 hours during walking hours.
MOBILITY ability to change and control body position	**1. Completely Immobile:** Does not make even slight changes in body extremity position without assistance.	**2. Very Limited:** Makes occasional slight changes in body or extremity position but unable to make frequent or significant changes independently.	**3. Slightly Limited:** Makes frequent though slight changes in body or extremity positions independently.	**4. No limitations:** Makes major and frequent changes in position without assistance.
NUTRITION usual food intake pattern	**1. Very Poor:** Never eats a complete meal. Rarely eats more than a third of any food offered. East 2 servings or less or protein (meat or dairy products) per day. Takes fluids poorly. Does not take a liquid dietary supplement. OR Is NPO and/or maintained on clear liquids or IVs for more than 5 days.	**2. Probably Inadequate:** Rarely eats a complete meal and generally eats only about half of any food offered. Protein intake includes only 3 servings of meat or dairy products per day. Occasionally will take a dietary supplement. OR Receives less than optimum amount of liquid diet or tube feeding.	**3. Adequate:** Eats over half most meals. Eats a total of 4 servings of protein (meat, dairy products) each day. Occasionally will refuse a meal, but will usually take a supplement if offered. OR Is on a tube feeding or TPN regimen that probably meets most of nutritional needs.	**4. Excellent:** Eats most of every meal. Never refuses a meal. Usually eats a total of 4 or more servings of meat and dairy products. Occasionally east between meals. Does not require supplementation.

Exhibit 6–2 continued

**FRICTION AND
SHEAR**

1. Problem:
Requires moderate to maximum assistance in moving. Complete lifting without sliding against sheets is impossible. Frequently slides down in bed or chair, requiring frequent repositioning with maximum assistance. Spasticity, contractors, or agitation leads to almost constant friction.

**2. Potential
Problem:**
Moves feebly or requires minimum assistance. During a move, skin probably slides to some extent against sheets, chair, restraints, or other devices. Maintains relatively good position in chair or bed most of the time but occasionally slides down.

**3. No Apparent
Problem:** Moves in bed and in chair independently and has sufficient muscle strength to lift up completely during move. Maintains good position in bed or chair at all times.

Exhibit 6–3 Nutritional Risk Screening Form

Name: _____ Pt #: _____ DOB: _____

Physician's Name: _____ Phone #: _____

Diagnosis: _____ Diet Order: _____

Height: _____   Weight: Current _____   1 month ago _____   6 months ago _____

NUTRITION RISK INDICATORS

Check/date all that apply.

Indicator	Criteria	
❑ Weight change from usual	❑ > 10-lb change in 3 months ❑ 5% weight change in 1 month	❑ BMI < 22
❑ High-risk diagnosis	❑ Hip fracture/replacement ❑ Pressure ulcer, wounds ❑ GI disease ❑ Dysphagia ❑ Other _____	❑ Pneumonia ❑ Cancer ❑ CHF ❑ COPD ❑ Depression ❑ CVA ❑ Diabetes ❑ HIV/AIDS ❑ Renal failure

❑ Complex diet order	❑ > 3 dietary modifications
	❑ Receiving medical nutritional
	  supplement
	❑ Transitioning from EN to oral, or
	  PN to EN
		❑ Tube feeding
		❑ Parenteral nutrition support

❑ Physical signs	❑ Poor skin turgor ❑ Dry mucous membranes ❑ Muscle wasting ❑ Weakness/tremors ❑ Psychosocial factors	❑ Edema ❑ Oral lesions ❑ Dull, dry, and/or brittle hair
❑ Psychosocial factors	❑ No caregiver in the home ❑ No transportation	❑ Limited mobility (inability to prepare food) ❑ Limited funds to buy food

❏ Other: _____

Signed: _____ Date: _____

NUTRITION RISK DETERMINATION

❏ Low risk (no indicators checked). Reassess in _____ days.
❏ Moderate risk (one indicator checked).
❏ High risk (two or more indicators checked).

INTERVENTIONS

❏ Initiate interdisciplinary care plan for _____
❏ Provide Ensure® Patient Starter Kit
❏ Request RD chart consult
❏ Request RD home referral

Signed: _____ Date: _____

The At-Risk Patient

Pressure Reduction

Refer to Medicare Part B Guidelines for Specialty Mattresses in the Home (Exhibit 6–4, page 107). Group 1 support surfaces may be used for prevention.

- air or foam overlays
- nonpowered mattress replacements

Wheelchair cushions should be fitted by patient need and reassessed periodically for efficiency. Avoid use of donut-style seat cushions.

Patient Movement

- Reposition the at-risk patient every two hours while in bed. Ideally adjust the schedule to best meet the patient's needs.
- Limit sitting intervals to two hours, with weight shifts every 15 minutes.
- Perform range-of-motion exercises daily.

Exhibit 6–4 Medicare Part B Guidelines for Specialty Mattresses in the Home

Patient qualifications are expressed in summary terms. For clarification and specific terms, contact your DMERC. Guidelines are subject to change without any notice.

GROUP 1

These products are overlays and nonpowered replacements. Patients should have at least one of these characteristics:

- immobility
- a pressure ulcer on the trunk or pelvis
- limited mobility plus one of the following:
  - incontinence
  - malnutrition
  - altered sensory perception
  - compromised circulatory status

GROUP 2

These products are low-air-loss or alternating pressure mattress replacements. Patients should have at least one of these characteristics:

- large or multiple Stage III or IV pressure ulcer(s) on the trunk or pelvis
- multiple Stage II pressure ulcers on the trunk or pelvis that have not improved within 30 days on a Group 1 product
- a requirement for a continuation of therapy from hospital or nursing home for recent ulcer, flap, or graft procedures (surgery within the past 60 days)

GROUP 3

These products are air-fluidized beds. Patients must have *all* of the following characteristics:

- Stage III or IV pressure ulcer on trunk or pelvis
- bedridden/severe immobility
- required institutionalization without air-fluidized bed
- physician order and monthly rectification
- care plan/assessment
- Group 2 product tried without success
- trained adult caregiver available

- Maintain good alignment.
- Use turn sheets and lifting devices.
- Use trapeze when indicated.
- Do not elevate the head of the bed over 30 degrees (may lead to shearing at sacrum).
- The heels should be floated off the bed surface at all times.

Nutrition

Nutritional assessment for the at-risk patient may include:

- albumin level
  - normal range = 3.5–5 g/dl (grams per deciliter)
  - mild depletion = 2.8–3.4 g/dl
  - moderate depletion = 2.4–2.7 g/dl
  - severe depletion < 2.1 g/dl
- Nutritional Risk Screening Form (Exhibit 6–3)
- 3-day intake diary
- weight loss (may be difficult to assess in bedbound patient due to lack of bed scales in the home)

For at-risk patients: (adapt to the individual needs of the patient)

- Increase intake (add supplements, high-protein milk, powdered milk, eggs, peanut butter, cheese).
- Increase caloric intake (small, frequent feedings, butter, creams, fats, sugars).
- Encourage fluids.
- Add multivitamin with minerals.

Consult a clinical dietitian as needed. See Chapter 4 for more information on nutrition.

Skin Care

Maintain clean, soft, supple skin.

Bathing

- Schedule baths based on patient need.
- Use mild soaps.
- Use moisturizers.

Incontinence

- Always evaluate for etiology and treat appropriately.
- Cleanse immediately using products designed for perineal care.
- Protect skin from the next episode of incontinence with the use of moisture barriers.
- Minimize use of diapers; use only when patient is out of bed.
- One open underpad on the bed should be sufficient when the patient is in bed.

Education

- Education must be patient-specific.
- Patient and caregiver must be active participants.
- Multidisciplinary approaches may be needed, including
  - physical therapy
  - occupational therapy
  - speech therapy
  - nutritional services
  - social services
- Instructions should be verbal and written, at the patient and caregiver's level of understanding (see Appendix 6–A, page 119).
- Patients and caregivers should provide demonstrations to show understanding of teaching provided and verbalize a willingness to follow through on the developed plan of care.
- Monitor, on all patients, any variance. For example, home care and skilled nursing facility acquired pressure ulcers should be logged, tracked, and reported in compliance with agency policy.

TIP Case management of at-risk patients is essential. Communication between the patient, caregiver, and staff involved is imperative, as is consistency with adherence to the developed plan of care.

TREATMENT CHOICES

Goals

- Prevent further breakdown.

- Reduce risk factors.
- Utilize appropriate topical therapy.
- Utilize appropriate adjunct therapy.

Pressure Reduction

Group 2 mattresses are for treatment only, not prevention. Group 2 mattresses are:

- mattress replacements
- alternating air or low-air-loss mattresses

Patients must meet certain criteria to qualify for reimbursement of the mattress cost.

Group 3 mattresses are air-fluidized therapy. Patients must meet criteria for reimbursement.

Patient Movement

Patients must not be positioned on a pressure ulcer. If there are no turning surfaces without breakdown, the patient must be turned hourly and must be on a Group 2 or 3 mattress.

Nutrition

Maintain adequate nutrition that is compatible with the individual's wishes or condition. Consult with a clinical dietitian. See Exhibit 6–3, pages 105–106.

Skin Care

Incontinence

Measures should be taken to avoid contamination of a wound from episodes of incontinence. Precautions include:

- occlusive dressings if indicated
- Foley catheters
- fecal incontinence devices
- bowel and bladder programs

Periwound Skin

Use protective skin barrier wipes.

Local Wound Treatment

- Cleanse or irrigate with normal saline.
- Choose the optimum category of wound product based on stage, location, and assessment of the wound.
- Refer to Topical Treatment (Chapter 5).

TIP Once a pressure ulcer has closed, the site remains extremely vulnerable to repeat breakdown. Aggressive measures are needed to prevent recurrence.

CASE STUDY

Mr. Brown is a 68-year-old male admitted to home care following a cerebral vascular accident with resultant left-sided paralysis and swallowing difficulties. He has an indwelling Foley catheter for neurogenic bladder and has occasionally been incontinent of stool. His Braden Scale score is 14, showing a moderate risk for skin breakdown. His wife, age 65, is a homemaker and a willing and able caregiver. One daughter lives nearby; a son lives two hours away. The home is considered clean, tidy, and adequate for care.

A multidisciplinary approach was taken to plan Mr. Brown's care. The RN case manager led the team. It included a physical therapist to assist/instruct in transfers and strengthening, an occupational therapist to instruct in maximizing resumption of activities of daily living, a speech therapist to assess and assist with swallowing problems, a social worker for community resources and respite care, and a home health aide to assist with personal care.

Medical equipment ordered included a hospital bed with a Group 1 mattress replacement, a trapeze, a bedside commode, a wheelchair, and a therapeutic foam seating cushion.

The RN instructed Mr. and Mrs. Brown in the importance of maintaining skin integrity through positioning, nutrition, and routine skin care. Together they constructed a schedule (see below) that was acceptable to all involved.

After two months of care and instructions, Mrs. Brown felt able to care for her spouse with a monthly visit from the RN to change the Foley and reassess the patient's status. She continued to have a home health aide three times weekly to assist with bathing and personal care (this also gave Mrs. Brown time to shop and tend to her needs).

Mr. Brown did not develop any pressure ulcers in a one-year period from the time of his admission to home care.

Mr. Brown's Schedule

8 AM	Up in wheelchair for breakfast
9 AM	Toileting regimen
10 AM	Bath:
	• Monday, Wednesday, Friday by home health aide
	• Tuesday & Thursday by spouse
	• Saturday & Sunday by daughter
11 AM	Bed, right side
Noon	Lunch, in bed with head of bed elevated
1 PM	Nap on left side
3:30 PM	Up in wheelchair to watch TV, weight shifts with each commercial break
5 PM	Dinner in wheelchair
6 PM	Toileting, then in recliner chair for reading or TV
9 PM	Bed, on back with head of bed not elevated over 30°, range- of-motion exercises performed
10 PM	Snack (high protein) with head of bed elevated
10:30 PM	Right side with pillow supports for back and knees
2:30 AM	Pillows removed, on back
6:30 AM	Draw sheet used to turn to left side, one small pillow for support

The AHCPR Pressure Ulcer Treatment Guidelines for the Patient were utilized in instructing the caregiver. (See Appendix 6–A.)

See Exhibit 6–5, page 113, for a teaching guide on the treatment and prevention of pressure ulcers.

Exhibit 6–5 Teaching Guide: Guide Specific to Treatment and Prevention of Pressure Ulcers

	Instructions Given (Date/Initials)	Demonstration or Review of Material (Date/Initials)	Return Demonstration or States Understanding (Date/Initials)
1. Identification of specific risk factors for pressure ulcer development			
2. Immobility, inactivity, and decreased sensory perception strategies			
a. Passive repositioning			
(1) Demonstrates one-person turning			
(2) Demonstrates two-person turning			
(3) Frequency of turning/ repositioning			
(4) Full shifts in position versus small shifts in position			
(5) Avoidance of 90° sidelying position, demonstrates 30° laterally inclined position			
(6) Passive range of motion exercises and frequency			
b. Pillow bridging			
(1) Use of pillows to protect heels			
(2) Pillows between bony prominences			
c. Pressure-reducing/relieving support surface			
(1) Management of support surface in use			
(2) Devices for sitting			
(3) Up in chair for _____ hour(s), _____ time(s) per day			
3. Nutrition strategies			
a. Provide adequate nutrition			
(1) Importance of adequate nutrition for wound healing			

Exhibit 6–5 continued

	Instructions Given (Date/Initials)	Demonstration or Review of Material (Date/Initials)	Return Demonstration or States Understanding (Date/Initials)
(2) Small frequent (six meals a day) high-calorie/high-protein meals			
(3) Nutritional supplements provided. Give _____ oz of _____ supplement _____ times per day.			
b. Provide adequate hydration			
(1) Eight 8-oz glasses of noncaffeine fluids per day unless contraindicated			
c. Provide vitamin/mineral supplements			
(1) Vitamin C, zinc, iron (Give as ordered.)			
4. Friction and shear strategies			
a. Use of turning and draw sheets			
b. Use of cornstarch, lubricants, pad protectors, thin film dressings, or hydrocolloid dressings over friction risk sites			
c. General skin care			
(1) Skin cleansing			
(2) Skin moisturizing (Use _____ product on _____ areas of skin, _____ times a day.)			
5. Moisture—incontinence management strategies			
a. Use of absorbent products			
(1) Pad when lying in bed			
b. Use of ointments, creams, and skin barriers prophylactically in perineal and perianal areas (Use _____ product on perineal/perianal areas of skin, _____ times a day.)			

Exhibit 6–5 continued

	Instructions Given (Date/Initials)	Demonstration or Review of Material (Date/Initials)	Return Demonstration or States Understanding (Date/Initials)
c. General skin care			
(1) Skin cleansing			
(a) Cleanser: _____			
(b) Soap: _____			
(c) Frequency: _____			
(2) Skin moisturizing (Use _____ product(s) on _____ areas of skin, _____ _____ times a day.)			
(3) Skin inspection daily			
6. Wound dressing care routine			
a. Wash hands, then remove old dressing and discard			
b. Clean wound with normal saline			
c. Apply primary dressing to wound			
d. Apply secondary dressing if appropriate			
e. Secure dressing with tape			
f. Universal precautions and dressing disposal			
g. Frequency of dressing changes			
7. When to notify the health care provider			
a. Signs and symptoms of wound infection (erythema, edema, pain, elevated temperature, change in exudate character or amount, discoloration in tissues surrounding wound)			
8. Importance of follow-up with health care provider			

Note: These guidelines must be individualized for each patient and caregiver.

REFERENCE

Stotts, N., and Cavanaugh, C. 1999. Assessing the patient with a wound. *Home Health Care Nurse* (17)1, 27–35.

BIBLIOGRAPHY

Ayello, E. A., and Draden, B. How and why to do pressure ulcer risk assessment. *Advances in Skin and Wound Care* 15(3), 125–132, May–June 2002.

Baharestani, M. 1999. Pressure ulcers in an age of managed care: A nursing perspective. *Ostomy/Wound Management* (45)5, 18–40.

Bergquist, S., and Frantz. R. 1999. Pressure ulcers in community-based older adults receiving home health care: Prevalence, incidence and associated risk factors. *Advanced Wound Care* 12, 339–351.

Blaszcyk, J. 1998. Make a difference: Standardize your heel care practice. *Ostomy/Wound Management* (44)5, 32–40.

Cali, T.G. et al. 1999. Pressure ulcer treatment: Examining selected costs of therapeutic failure. *Advanced Wound Care* 12 (supplement 2), 8–11.

Coverage and payment policy for support sufaces. In *DMERC Provider Reimbursement Manual updates and bulletins.* Indianapolis, IN: Administar Federalist; September 1995, December 1995, and March 1996.

Dudek, S. 2000. Malnutrition in hospitals: Who's assessing what patients eat? *American Journal of Nursing* (100)4, 36–43.

Egger, C. 1997. Monitoring wound healing in the home health arena. *Advanced Wound Care* (10)5, 54–57.

Haalboom, J. 1999. Risk-assessment tools in the prevention of pressure ulcers. *Ostomy/Wound Management* (45)2, 20–34.

Maklebust, J., and Sieggreen, M. 1996. *Pressure ulcers: Guidelines for prevention and nursing management,* 2d ed. Springhouse, PA: Springhouse Corp.

National Pressure Ulcer Advisory Panel. 1989. *Pressure ulcers: Incidence, economics, risk assessment. Consensus Development Conference Statement.* West Dundee, IL: S-N Publications, 3–4.

Panel for the Prediction and Prevention of Pressure Ulcers. 1992. *Pressure ulcers in adults: Prediction and prevention, Clinical Practice Guideline No. 3.* AHCPR Publication No. 92-0047. Rockville, MD: Agency for Health Care Policy and Research, U.S. Public Health Service, U.S. Department of Health and Human Services.

Pieper, B. 1998. Pressure ulcer management: Making prevention a more attainable goal. *Advance for Nurse Practitioners,* October, 55–58.

Pieper, B. et al. 1997. Presence of pressure ulcer prevention methods used among patients considered at risk versus those considered not at risk. *Journal of Wound Ostomy and Continence Nursing* 24, 191–199.

Provo, B. et al. 1997. Practice versus knowledge when it comes to pressure ulcer prevention. *Journal of Wound Ostomy and Continence Nursing* 24, 265–269.

Richardson, G. et al. 1998. Nursing assessment: Impact on type and cost of interventions to prevent pressure ulcers. *Journal of Wound Ostomy and Continence Nursing* 25, 273–280.

Van Rijswijk, L., and Braden, B. 1999. Pressure ulcer patient and wound assessment: An AHCPR clinical practice guideline update. *Ostomy/Wound Management* 45 (Suppl 1A), 565–675.

Patient Guide: AHCPR Pressure Ulcer Treatment Guidelines for the Patient

A pressure sore is serious. It must not be ignored. With proper treatment, most pressure sores will heal. Healing depends on many things: your general health, diet, relieving pressure on the sore, and careful cleaning and dressing of the sore. Share this handout with your family members and caregivers. By working with health care professionals and following these guidelines, you and your caregiver can better treat pressure sores and prevent new ones.

This handout will help you and your caregiver care for pressure sores. It also gives basic information about preventing new sores.

This handout gives the steps essential to helping a pressure sore heal. Although not all steps apply to everyone, it is important that you:

- Learn how to prevent and treat pressure sores.
- Ask questions if you do not understand.
- Explain your needs and concerns.
- Know what is best for you.
- Be active in your care.

TREATMENT

Healing a pressure sore is a team effort. A team of health care professionals will work with you to prepare a treatment plan. Your team may include doctors, nurses, dietitians, social workers, pharmacists, and occupational and physical therapists. However, you and your caregiver are the most important team members. Feel free to ask questions or share concerns with other team members.

Your Role

You and your caregiver need to:

- Know your roles in the treatment program.
- Learn how to perform the care.
- Know what to report to the physician or nurse.
- Know how to tell if the treatment works.
- Help change the treatment plan when needed.
- Know what questions you want to ask.
- Get answers you understand.

Treatment Plan

To develop a treatment plan that meets your needs, the physician or nurse must know about

- your general health
- illnesses that might slow healing (such as diabetes or hardening of the arteries)
- prescription or over-the-counter medicines you take
- the emotional support and physical assistance available from family, friends, and others

Your physician or nurse will perform a physical exam and check the condition of your pressure sore to decide how to care for it. If you have had a pressure sore before, tell the physician or nurse what helped it heal and what didn't help.

Your emotional health is also important. Be sure to share information about stresses in your life as well as health beliefs and practices. This will help your care team design a treatment plan that meets your personal needs.

The treatment plan will be based on the results of your physical exam, health history, personal circumstances, and the condition of the sore (how it looks). This plan will include specific instructions for

- taking pressure off the sore
- caring for the pressure sore by cleaning the wound, removing dead tissue and debris, and dressing or bandaging the area to protect it while it heals
- aiding healing by making sure you get enough calories, protein, vitamins, and minerals

Note to Caregivers

Although patients should be as active in their care as possible, you may need to provide much or all of their care. As a result, you may find you have questions or problems. If so, ask for help. Call physicias, nurses, and other professionals for answers and other support.

Remember that patients who must be in a bed or chair for long periods don't have to get pressure sores. Pressure sores can be prevented, and sores that have formed can be healed.

Helping Pressure Sores Heal

Healing pressure sores depends on three principles: pressure relief, care of the sore, and good nutrition.

PRESSURE RELIEF

Pressure sores form when there is constant pressure on certain parts of the body. Long periods of unrelieved pressure cause or worsen pressure sores and slow healing once a sore has formed. Taking pressure off the sore is the first step toward healing.

Pressure sores usually form on parts of the body over bony prominences (such as hips and heels) that bear weight when you sit or lie down

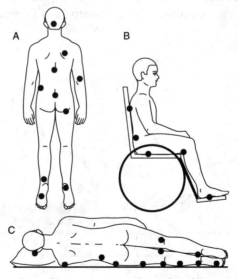

Figure 6–A1. Pressure Points. Dots show pressure points when lying on back (A), when sitting (B), and when lying on side (C).

for a long time. Figure 6–A1 shows "pressure points" where sores often form.

You can relieve or reduce pressure by

- using special surfaces to support your body
- putting your body in certain positions
- changing positions often

Support Surfaces

Support surfaces are special beds, mattresses, mattress overlays, or seat cushions that support your body in bed or in a chair. These surfaces reduce or relieve pressure. By relieving pressure, you can help pressure sores heal and prevent new ones from forming.

You can get different kinds of support surfaces. The best kind depends on your general health, if you are able to change positions, your body build, and the condition of your sore. You and your physician or nurse can choose the surface best for you.

One way to see if a support surface reduces pressure enough is for the caregiver to do a "hand check" under the person (Figure 6–A2). The caregiver places his or her hand under the support surface, beneath the pressure point, with the palm up and fingers flat. If there is less than one inch of support surface between the pressure point of the body and the caregiver's hand, the surface does not give enough support. If you need more support, your physician or nurse will recommend a different support surface.

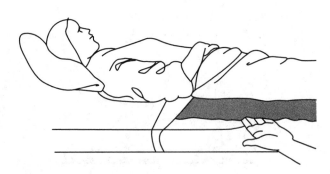

Figure 6–A2 Hand Check to Assess Pressure Relief. Slide hand (palm up and fingers flat) under support surface, just under pressure point. Do not flex fingers.

Caregivers should know that pressure sores are often painful, and a hand check may increase pain. Caregivers should ask if it will be okay to do a hand check, which should be done as gently as possible.

Good Body Positions

Your position is important to relieving pressure on the sore and preventing new ones. You need to switch positions whether you are in a bed or a chair.

In Bed

Follow these guidelines:

- Do not lie on the pressure sore. Use foam pads or pillows to relieve pressure on the sore, as shown in Figure 6–A3.

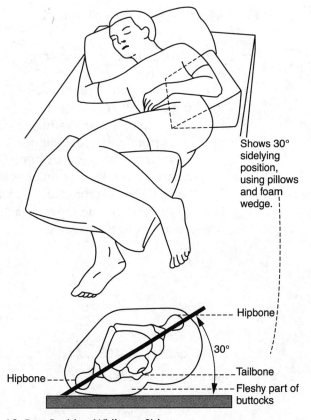

Shows 30°
sidelying
position,
using pillows
and foam
wedge.

Hipbone

30°

Hipbone

Tailbone

Fleshy part of
buttocks

Figure 6–A3 Best Position While on Side.

- Change position at least every two hours.
- Do not rest directly on your hip bone when lying on your side. A 30- degree, sidelying position is best (Figure 6–A3).
- When lying on your back, keep your heels up off the bed by placing a thin foam pad or pillow under your legs from midcalf to ankle (Figure 6–A4). The pad or pillow should raise the heels just enough so a piece of paper can be passed between them and the bed. Do not place the pad or pillow directly under the knee when on your back, because this could reduce blood flow to your lower leg.

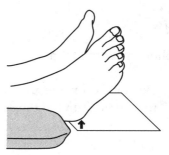

Figure 6–A4 Keep Heels off Bed.

- Do not use donut-shaped (ring) cushions—they reduce blood flow to tissue.
- Use pillows or small foam pads to keep knees and ankles from touching each other.
- Raise the head of the bed as little as possible. Raise it no more than 30 degrees from horizontal (Figure 6–A5). If you have other health problems (such as respiratory ailments) that are improved by sitting up, ask your doctor or nurse which positions are best.
- Use the upright position during meals to prevent choking. The head of the bed can be moved back to a lying or semireclining position one hour after eating.

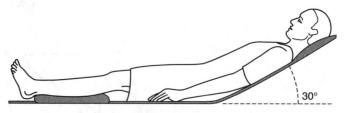

Figure 6–A5 Head of Bed Raised 30 Degrees.

In a Chair or Wheelchair

When sitting, you should have good posture and be able to keep upright in the chair or wheelchair (Figure 6–A6). A good position will allow you to move more easily and help prevent new sores.

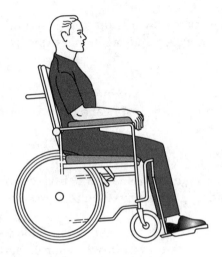

Figure 6–A4 Best Position While Sitting

For your specific needs, use cushions designed to relieve pressure on sitting surfaces. Even if pressure can be relieved with cushions, your position should be changed every hour. Remember to

- Avoid sitting directly on the pressure sore.
- Keep the top of your thighs horizontal and your ankles in a comfortable, "neutral" position on the floor or footrest (Figure 6–A6). Rest your elbows, forearms, and wrists on arm supports.
- If you cannot move yourself, have someone help you change your position at least every hour. If you can move yourself, shifting your weight every 15 minutes is even better.
- If your position in a chair cannot be changed, have someone help you back to bed so you can change position.
- Do not use donut-shaped or ring cushions because they reduce blood flow to tissue.

Changing Positions

Change your body position often—at least every hour while seated in a chair and at least every two hours while lying in bed. A written turning schedule or a turn clock (with positions written next to times) may help you and your caregiver remember turning times and positions. You may want to set a kitchen timer.

Be sure your plan works for you. It should consider your skin's condition, personal needs and preferences, and your comfort level.

PRESSURE SORE CARE

The second principle of healing is proper care of the sore. The three aspects of care are

- cleaning
- removing dead tissue and debris (debridement)
- dressing (bandaging) the pressure sore

Pressure sore care is summarized in Table 6–A1, page 127. You should know about sore care even if only your caregiver is caring for the sore. Knowing about your care will help you make informed decisions about it.

Cleaning

Pressure sores heal best when they are clean. They should be free of dead tissue (which may look like a scab), excess fluid draining from the sore, and other debris. If not, healing can be slowed, and infection can result.

A health care professional will show you and your caregiver how to clean and/or rinse the pressure sore. Clean the sore each time dressings are changed.

Cleaning usually involves rinsing, or "irrigating," the sore. Loose material may also be gently wiped away with a gauze pad. It is important to use the right equipment and methods for cleaning the sore. Tissue that is healing can be hurt if too much force is used when rinsing. Cleaning may be ineffective if too little force is used.

Use only cleaning solutions recommended by a health care professional. Usually saline is best for rinsing the pressure sore. Saline can be bought at a drug store or made at home (see Table 6–A2, page 128).

Caution: Sometimes water supplies become contaminated. If the health department warns against drinking the water, use saline from the drug store or use bottled water to make saline for cleaning sores.

Table 6–A1 Basic Steps of Pressure Sore Care

Task	Steps
Prepare	1. Wash hands with soap and water.
	2. Get supplies: saline; irrigation equipment (syringe or other device, basin, large plastic bag); dressings and tape; disposable plastic gloves and small plastic (sandwich) bag; towel; glasses, goggles, and plastic apron (optional).
	3. Move patient into comfortable position.
	4. Place large plastic bag on bed to protect bed linen.
Remove dressing	1. Place hand into small plastic bag (Figure 6–A7).
	2. Grasp old dressing with bag-covered hand and pull off dressing.
	3. Turn bag inside out over the old dressing.
	4. Close the bag tightly before throwing it away.
Irrigate the sore	1. Put on disposable plastic gloves. (Wear glasses or goggles and plastic apron if drainage might splash.)
	2. Fill syringe or other device with saline.
	3. Place basin under pressure sore to catch drainage.
	4. Hold irrigation device 1 to 6 inches from sore and spray it with saline. Use enough force to remove dead tissue and old drainage, but not enough to damage new tissue.
	5. Carefully remove basin so fluid doesn't spill.
	6. Dry the skin surrounding the sore by patting skin with soft, clean towel.
	7. After assessing and dressing the sore, remove gloves by pulling them inside out. Throw away gloves properly.
Assess the sore	1. Assess healing. As sore heals, it will slowly become smaller and drain less. New tissue at the bottom of the sore is light red or pink and looks lumpy and glossy. Do not disturb this tissue.
	2. Tell health care provider if the sore is larger, drainage increases, the sore is infected, or there are no signs of healing in 2 to 4 weeks.
Dress the sore	Place a new dressing over the sore as instructed by the physician or nurse. Remember to:
	• Use dressings only once.
	• Keep dressings in the original package or other closed plastic package.
	• Store dressings in a clean, dry place.
	• Throw out the entire package if any dressings get wet, contaminated, or dirty.
	• Wash your hands before touching clean dressings.
	• Do not touch packaged dressings once you touch the sore.

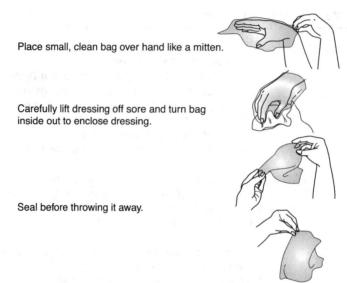

Place small, clean bag over hand like a mitten.

Carefully lift dressing off sore and turn bag inside out to enclose dressing.

Seal before throwing it away.

Figure 6–A7 Plastic Bag Method of Removing Bandages.

Table 6–A2 Recipe for Making Saline (Salt Water)

1. Use 1 gallon of distilled water or boil 1 gallon of tap water for 5 minutes. Do not use well water or sea water. Be sure storage container and mixing utensil are clean (boiled).
2. Add 8 teaspoons of table salt to the distilled or boiled water.
3. Mix the solution well until the salt is completely dissolved.

Note: Cool to room temperature before using. This solution can be stored at room temperature in a tightly covered glass or plastic bottle for up to 1 week.

Do not use antiseptics such as hydrogen peroxide or iodine. They can damage sensitive tissue and prevent healing.

Cleansing methods are usually effective in keeping sores clean. However, in some cases, other methods will be needed to remove dead tissue.

Removing Dead Tissue and Debris

Dead tissue in the pressure sore can delay healing and lead to infection. Removing dead tissue is often painful. You may want to take pain-relieving medicine 30 to 60 minutes before these procedures.

Under supervision of health care professionals, dead tissue and debris can be removed in several ways:

- rinsing (to wash away loose debris)
- wet-to-dry dressings. In this special method, wet dressings are put on and allowed to dry. Dead tissue and debris are pulled off when the dry dressing is taken off. This method is only used to remove dead tissue; it is never used on a clean wound.
- enzyme medications to dissolve dead tissue only
- special dressings left in place for several days help the body's natural enzymes dissolve dead tissue slowly. This method should not be used if the sore is infected. With infected sores, a faster method for removing dead tissue and debris should be used.

Qualified health care professionals may use surgical instruments to cut away dead tissue.

Based on the person's general health and the condition of the sore, the physician or nurse will recommend the best method for removing dead tissue.

Choosing and Using Dressings

Choosing the right dressings is important to pressure sore care. The physician or nurse will consider the location and condition of the pressure sore when recommending dressings.

The most common dressings are gauze (moistened with saline), film (see-through), and hydrocolloid (moisture- and oxygen-retaining) dressings. Gauze dressings must be moistened often with saline and changed at least daily. If they are not kept moist, new tissue will be pulled off when the dressing is removed.

Unless the sore is infected, film or hydrocolloid dressings can be left on for several days to keep in the sore's natural moisture.

The choice of dressing is based on

- the type of material that will best aid healing
- how often dressings will need to be changed
- whether the sore is infected

In general, the dressing should keep the sore moist and the surrounding skin dry. As the sore heals, a different type of dressing may be needed.

Storing and Caring for Dressings

Clean (rather than sterile) dressings usually can be used, if they are kept clean and dry. There is no evidence that using sterile dressings is better than using clean dressings. However, contamination between patients can occur in hospitals and nursing homes. When clean dressings are used in institutions, procedures that prevent cross-contamination should be followed carefully.

At home, clean dressings may also be used. Carefully follow the methods given below on how to store, care for, and change dressings.

To keep dressings clean and dry:

- Store dressings in their original packages (or in other protective, closed plastic packages) in a clean, dry place.
- Wash hands with soap and water before touching clean dressings.
- Take dressings from the box only when they will be used.
- Do not touch the packaged dressing once the sore has been touched.
- Discard the entire package if any dressings become wet or dirty.

Changing Dressings

Ask your physician or nurse to show you how to remove dressings and put on new ones. If possible, he or she should watch you change the dressings at least once.

Ask for written instructions if you need them. Discuss any problems or questions about changing dressings with the physician or nurse.

Wash your hands with soap and water before and after each dressing change. Use each dressing only once. You should check to be sure the dressing stays in place when changing positions. After the used dressing is removed, it must be disposed of safely to prevent the spread of germs that may be on dressings.

Using Plastic Bags for Removal

A small plastic bag (such as a sandwich bag) can be used to lift the dressing off the pressure sore (Figure 6–A7). Seal the bag before throwing it away. If you use gloves, throw them away after each use.

GOOD NUTRITION

Good nutrition is the third principle of healing. Eating a balanced diet will help your pressure sore heal and prevent new sores from forming.

You and your physician, dietitian, or nurse should review any other medical conditions you have (such as diabetes or kidney problems) before designing a special diet.

Weigh yourself weekly. If you find you cannot eat enough food to maintain your weight or if you notice a sudden increase or decrease, you may need a special diet and vitamin supplements. You may need extra calories as part of a well-balanced diet.

Tell your physician or nurse about any weight change. An unplanned weight gain or loss of 10 pounds or more in six months should be looked into.

PAIN AND INFECTION

Even if you care for your pressure sore properly, problems may come up. Pain and infection are two such problems. Pain can make it hard to move or to participate in care. Infection can slow healing.

Managing Pain

You may feel pain in or near the pressure sore. Tell your physician or nurse if you do. Covering the sore with a dressing or changing your body position may lessen the pain.

If you feel pain during cleaning of the pressure sore or during dressing changes, medicine may help. It may be over-the-counter or prescription medicine. Take medicine to relieve pain 30 to 60 minutes before these procedures to give it time to work. Tell your physician or nurse if your pain medicine does not work.

Treating Infection

Healing may slow if the sore becomes infected. Infection from the sore can spread to surrounding tissue (cellulitis), to underlying bone (osteomyelitis), or throughout the body (sepsis). These serious complications demand immediate medical attention. **If you notice any of the signs of infection as described in Table 6–A3, page 132, call your physician right away.**

Table 6–A3 Signs of Infection

Infected Sore	Widespread Infection
Thick green or yellow drainage	Fever or chills
Foul odor	Weakness
Redness or warmth around sore	Confusion or difficulty concentrating
Tenderness of surrounding area	Rapid heartbeat
Swelling	

CHECKING YOUR PROGRESS

A health care professional should check your pressure sore regularly. How often depends on how well the sore is healing. Generally, a pressure sore should be checked weekly.

Examining the Sore

The easiest time to check pressure sores is after cleaning. Signs of healing include decreased size and depth of the sore and less drainage. You should see signs of healing in two to four weeks. Infected sores may take longer to heal.

Signs to Report

Tell your physician or nurse if:

- The pressure sore is larger or deeper.
- More fluid drains from the sore.
- The sore does not begin in heal in two to four weeks.
- You see signs of infection (Table 6–A3).

Also report if:

- You cannot eat a well-balanced diet.
- You have trouble following any part of the treatment plan.
- Your general health becomes worse.

Changing the Treatment Plan

If any of these signs exist, you and your health care professional may need to change the treatment plan. Depending on your needs, these factors may be changed:

- support surfaces
- how often you change how you sit or lie
- methods of cleaning and removing dead tissue
- type of dressing
- nutrition
- infection treatment

Other Treatment Choices

If sores do not heal, your physician may recommend electrotherapy. A very small electrical current is used to stimulate healing in this procedure. This is a fairly new treatment for pressure sores. Proper equipment and trained personnel may not always be available.

If your pressure sore is large or deep, or if it does not heal, surgery may be needed to repair damaged tissue. You and your physician can discuss possible surgery.

CARE OF HEALTHY SKIN

Having healthy skin is important to preventing future pressure sores. Healthy skin is less likely to be damaged and heals faster than skin in poor condition.

You can help prevent new pressure sores while helping to heal the ones you have. To improve your skin's health:

- Bathe when needed for cleanliness and comfort.
- Use mild soap and warm (not hot) water.
- Apply moisturizers (such as skin lotions) to keep skin from becoming too dry.

Inspect your skin at least once a day for redness or color changes or for sores. Pay special attention to pressure points where pressure sores can form (Figure 6–A1).

Skin problems can also result from bladder or bowel leakage (urinary or fecal incontinence). If you have these problems, ask your physician or nurse for help. If the leakage cannot be controlled completely, you should:

- Clean your skin as soon as it becomes soiled.
- Use a protective cream or ointment on the skin to protect it from wetness.

- Use incontinence pads and/or briefs to absorb wetness away from the skin.

For more detailed information about how to prevent pressure sores, ask for a copy of *Preventing Pressure Ulcers: Patient Guide*. To order, see the information below.

FOR MORE INFORMATION

Information in this handout is based on *Treatment of Pressure Ulcers, Clinical Practice Guideline*, No. 15. It was developed by a nonfederal panel sponsored by the Agency for Healthcare Research and Quality (AHRQ), formerly known as the Agency for Health Care Policy and Research (AHCPR), an agency of the Public Health Service. Other guidelines on common health problems are available, and more are being developed.

Four other patient guides are available from AHRQ that may be of interest to those at risk for or who have pressure sores and for their caregivers:

- *Preventing Pressure Ulcers: Patient Guide* gives detailed information about how to prevent pressure sores (AHCPR Publication No. 92-0048).
- *Urinary Incontinence in Adults: Patient Guide* describes why people lose urine when they don't want to and how that can be treated (AHCPR Publication No. 92-0040).
- *Pain Control after Surgery: Patient Guide* explains different types of pain treatment and how to work with physicians and nurses to prevent or relieve pain (AHCPR Publication No. 92-0021).
- *Depression Is a Treatable Illness: Patient Guide* discusses major depressive disorders, which can be successfully treated with the help of a health care professional (AHCPR Publication No. 93-0053).

For more information about these and other guidelines, or to get more copies of this handout, call (800) 358-9295, or write to:

Publications Clearinghouse
P.O. Box 8547
Silver Spring, MD 20907

BE ACTIVE IN YOUR CARE

If you understand the basic ideas of pressure relief, sore care, and good nutrition, you can take the steps needed to heal pressure sores and prevent new ones. Not all steps apply to every person. The best program will be based on your needs and the condition of your sores.

Be sure to:

- Ask questions.
- Explain your needs, wants, and concerns.
- Understand what is being done and why.
- Know what is best for you. Discuss what you can do to prevent and treat pressure sores—at home, in the hospital, or in the nursing home.

Being active in your care can mean better care.

ADDITIONAL RESOURCES

The following organizations offer a variety of resources for people concerned about pressure sores.

Booklets and Information for Patients, Caregivers, and Families Providing Care at Home

National Pressure Ulcer Advisory Panel (NPUAP)
12100 sunset Hills Rd.
Reston, VA 20190
Phone: (703) 464-4849; Fax (703) 435-4390
Contact: Robin M. Turner, Executive Director
E-mail: npuap@npuap.org

Information about Nutrition

National Center for Nutrition and Dietetics (NCND) Consumer Hotline, call (800) 366-1655.

U.S. Department of Health and Human Services Public Health Service

Agency for Health Care Research and Quality
Executive Office Center
Suite 501, 2101 East Jefferson Street
Rockville, MD 20852

CHAPTER 7

Arterial Ulcers

Julie Phelps Maloy

Arterial ulcers, usually located on the distal lower extremity, can be either acute or chronic. They have a round, punched out shape and a pale wound bed. They indicate a severe reduction or elimination of oxygenated blood flow to the leg or foot that has resulted in tissue ischemia and/or necrosis (Figure 7–1; Color Plate 14). The lack of oxygen to the tissue causes leg and/or foot pain for the patient. It is important to determine the type of pain the patient is experiencing. Is it burning, aching, or cramping? Is the pain constant or intermittent? Pain that is exercise-induced is referred to as intermittent claudication. Rest pain can be an indication of a threatened limb (Siegel 1998, 125). Some estimate approximately 21 percent of all lower extremity ulcers have some form of arterial involvement. Precipitating factors include diabetes, smoking, hypertension, and hypercholesterolemia (Rubano & Kerstein 1998, 147). The precipitating event leading to the ulceration is not always known but can result from progressive vessel occlusion or from trauma that leads to an increase in oxygen demands. Arterial disease and tissue ischemia set the stage, trauma occurs, and an ulcer results. Topical treatments are always important in chronic wound care; however, in ischemic ulcers, increased blood flow to the area through surgical intervention is the only effective way to heal the ulcer. Complications include infection, gangrene, and death. It is extremely important for the nurse to know if there is arterial involvement in a lower extremity ulcer (Figure 7–2; Color Plate 15). Without understanding the underlying cause of the ulcer, frustration results for the nurse and probable complications for the patient.

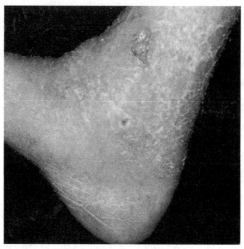

Figure 7–1 Arterial Ulcers. Note dry, flaky skin and absence of hair.
Clinical Objectives:
(1) Protect
(2) Clean
(3) Provide moisture cautiously
(4) Provide comfort.
See Color Plate 14.

ETIOLOGY

Arterial ulcers result from lack of blood supply, which can stem from several factors:

- atherosclerosis is the most common cause. Plaque forms on the walls of the arteries, causing a narrowing of the lumen and decreased blood flow. Plaque formation can lead to thrombosis, embolization, and ischemia.
- arterial embolism, when the body has no time to develop collateral circulation to compensate with resulting ischemia
- vasospastic disease (e.g., Raynaud's disease)
- trauma (open and/or closed injuries)
- diabetes mellitus

ASSESSMENT

Risk Factors

- hypertension

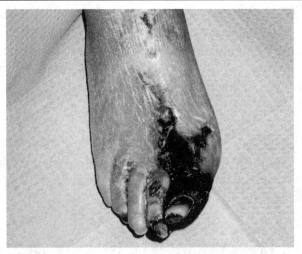

Figure 7–2 Ischemic Foot with Gangrene. Do not initiate topical treatment. Notify physician of status and any changes immediately.
See Color Plate 15.

- smoking
- diabetes mellitus
- hyperlipidemia
- male gender (males are more at risk than females)
- history of angina, myocardial infarction, or cerebrovascular accident

Clinical Signs

(See Appendix A and Appendix B at the end of this book for comparison charts with venous insufficiency, arterial insufficiency, and peripheral neuropathy.) (Holloway 1997, 158–172)

Wound

- uniform wound edges, a punched out appearance
- small in size but can be superficial or deep
- pale wound bed (due to the lack of oxygenated blood in the area) can also be gray or yellow with no new tissue
- limited or no surrounding inflammation
- minimal drainage
- necrosis (frequently present)
- loss of hair at the ankle or foot
- surrounding skin can appear shiny and tight

Location

Arterial ulcers are commonly found on the distal extremity. They can be above the malleoli; however, they are frequently found below, on the toe joints and/or lateral border of the foot. Trauma from footwear is a frequent cause of the ulcer formation.

Pain

- burning, cramping, or weariness located in the calf, thigh, buttocks, or foot
- located in foot when resting, particularly at night, indicating severe occlusion and a threatened limb
- increases with leg elevation
- increases with walking due to a lack of oxygen delivery to the working leg muscles (intermittent claudication) and can diminish within one to five minutes after the exertion is stopped
- usually focused distal to the point of occlusion in the vessel
- can be masked in the diabetic patient due to neuropathy
- can sometimes be relieved by a dependent leg position

Other Clinical Signs

- pallor of extremity on elevation
- dependent rubor of the extremity
- thickened, yellow, fragile nails
- pulses palpable or not palpable in the dorsalis pedis and posterior tibialis
  - dorsalis pedis: Use the second and third fingers to palpate the pulse on the dorsum of the foot. Place your thumb on the plantar surface of the foot to steady your hand. Use a light touch to avoid occluding the artery.
  - posterior tibialis: Palpate lightly posterior to the medial malleolus using the second and third fingers. Place your thumb on the lateral malleolus.
- foot cool or cold to touch
- absence of hair on the leg
- history of trauma to the foot or leg

Complications

- wound infection (Local signs can include erythema, edema, warmth, induration, increased pain, and purulent and/or an increase in wound exudate.)
- gangrene
- amputation
- death

TREATMENT CHOICES

Goal

To establish adequate circulation to the affected area (Ulcers associated with ischemia heal when the blood supply is reestablished.)

Diagnostics

Several systems can be used to confirm and locate perfusion problems.

- Noninvasive studies of the arterial system can be performed using an ultrasonic Doppler to determine the ankle-brachial index (ABI) (Falanga 1997, 169–170). (Exhibit 7–1, page 142)
  - A normal ABI is considered to be 0.9–1.1.
  - Claudication can occur between 0.5 and 0.6.
  - Tissue loss and rest pain (signaling a threatened limb) can occur at <0.5.

Most consider an ABI to be invalid in a diabetic patient. The increased atherosclerosis with resulting calcified vessels may cause a falsely elevated ABI.

- Segmental pressures help locate the site or sites of occlusion by a decrease in the pressure.
- Vascular laboratories can do transcutaneous oxygen measurements (tcpO$_2$) to help determine the degree of microvascular perfusion.
  - A reading of 20 mm Hg indicates that the ulcer will not heal.
  - A reading of >30 mm Hg indicates that healing can occur. Readings are not valid in the presence of a wound infection.

Exhibit 7–1 Ankle-Brachial Index

Definition: An ankle-brachial index (ABI) is a noninvasive Doppler test for determining the presence and severity of arterial occlusive disease by calculating the ratio of the systolic pressure at the ankle to the systolic pressure in the brachial artery in the arm (Siegel 1998, 129; Steed 1997, 173).

EQUIPMENT

1. Doppler probe (ultrasound stethoscope)

2. blood pressure cuff

   • Make sure the cuff size is appropriate for the arm size. A cuff that is too short or too narrow can give falsely high readings. The inflatable bladder of the cuff should have a width of about 40 percent of the upper arm circumference. The length of the bladder should be about 80 percent of the arm circumference.

   • A regular cuff on an obese arm can give a falsely high reading (Bickley & Hockelman 1999, 291).

3. ultrasound gel

PROCEDURE (Morison et al. 1997, 198–199)

1. The patient should lie flat for 15–20 minutes before obtaining pressure readings.

2. Apply the blood pressure cuff around the patient's arm, and apply ultrasound gel over the brachial pulse.

3. Hold the Doppler probe at a 45 degree angle, and place it over the brachial pulse.

4. When a good signal is obtained, inflate the cuff until the signal disappears and gradually deflate until the sound returns. The first sound heard is the systolic brachial pressure. Repeat in the other arm. Use the higher reading to calculate ABI.

5. Apply the cuff just above the ankle. Palpate the posterior tibial or dorsalis pedis pulse. Apply ultrasound gel.

6. Repeat steps 3 and 4.

7. $\text{ABI} = \dfrac{\text{ankle systolic pressure}}{\text{brachial systolic pressure}}$

INTERPRETATION

The ABI can be falsely elevated in those who have diabetes because there can be calcification of the inner layer of the arteries preventing the cuff from successfully compressing the arteries.

There are slight variations depending on the resource. Generally,

continues

Exhibit 7-1 continued

- 0.8–1.0 indicates that compression is an option for treatment: there is little or no arterial disease. (Some authorities will compress with 0.7.)

- If ABI equals 0.5–0.8, refer to a vascular specialist. The patient may be experiencing intermittent claudication. Compression is not indicated as a treatment option.

- At ≤ 0.5, refer to a vascular specialist. This is a threatened limb. Compression is contraindicated.

CASE STUDY

Systolic Doppler Pressures

	Brachial	Dorsalis Pedis	Posterior Tibial
Right	90	50	40
Left	100	0	100

Note: Always use the highest brachial pressure and the highest ankle pressure to calculate the ABI.

ABI = 50/100 = 0.5 in the right lower extremity; the highest ankle pressure is 50. Using the highest brachial pressure (which is the left arm), divide the 50 by 100, which equals 0.5.

ABI = 100/100 = 1.0 in the left lower extremity; the highest ankle pressure is 100. Using the left arm pressure again, divide the 100 at the ankle by the 100 brachial pressure, which equals 1.0.

Surgical Intervention for Revascularization

Indications include rest pain, ischemic ulceration, and gangrene. This disease is progressive; without surgery or with unsuccessful surgery, gangrene and amputation can occur within a relatively short period of time (from a few weeks to a few months).

Medical Management

Nonsurgical candidates require good wound care and patient education. Pentoxiphylline (Trental®) is used with some patients who are not experiencing resting pain. (There is controversy on its value for these patients.) Nurses should recognize that this is a progressive condition that can advance either slowly or rapidly.

Local Wound Management

- Clean the wound with normal saline or a commercially prepared wound cleanser.
- Removing eschar from heels and toes that have no symptoms of infection, leakage of exudate, or odor increases the opportunity for infection and can quickly lead to an amputation due to already compromised blood supply to the area. Refer to the reference list at the end of this chapter for further information on this subject.
- Select a dressing that supports realistic healing goals for the wound. Refer to Chapter 5, Wound Treatments, for information on topical dressings.

TIPS
- Consider the whole patient and the etiology. It is easy to get caught up in wanting the wound to heal with topical treatments and to forget the true cause of the ulcer.
- Explain the etiology to the patient along with signs and symptoms of complications.
- Without revascularization, the wound will usually become a chronic non-healing wound.

PREVENTION

Patient Education

(See Appendix 7–A, page 149).
- Provide information on the underlying cause of the ulceration(s).
- Reinforce dietary/blood sugar control for the diabetic patient.
- Stress the importance of cessation of smoking.
- Stress weight control and a mild exercise program (both for weight control and to build collateral circulation). Recommend a low-fat diet.
- Educate about blood pressure management (include a referral to stress reduction/management classes), if appropriate.
- Provide pharmacologic education on drug interactions and reactions for patients on medication.
- Explain that support stockings and compression are contraindicated because they further constrict the arteries.

- In regard to foot care, instruct the patient to
  - Wash, dry, and lubricate feet daily.
  - Check for cracks and reddened areas—report any cracks or sores to the physician.
  - Check the inside of each shoe before inserting the foot.
  - Avoid walking barefoot.
  - Have nail care done by a professional such as a podiatrist.
  - Wear correctly fit shoes, preferably fit by an orthodist or pedorthist.
- Educate the patient to signs and symptoms of complications along with what to do should they occur (including when to contact the physician and/or go to the emergency department). Complications include
  - increase in pain from intermittent claudication to resting pain
  - infection
  - increasing wound necrosis
  - gangrene

CASE STUDY

Sam Shell was referred to your agency from his physician's office. He is homebound with a painful, nonhealing ulcer of the left foot located slightly above the outer malleolus (ankle). His medical history includes recently diagnosed diabetes mellitus, managed by diet, and coronary heart disease. He is 65 years old, 5 feet 10 inches tall, and weighs 243 pounds. He quit smoking 4 years ago when he had coronary bypass surgery. He is a retired truck driver.

Sam tells you he bumped his leg on his lawn mower several months ago, and he hasn't been able to get the ulcer to heal. Recently, it has become larger. His treatment includes cleansing with hydrogen peroxide followed by the application of an antibiotic cream. He keeps it covered with a bandage. Sam tells you he used to spend more time in his yard, but now he only walks around his house because his legs and buttocks hurt when he walks very far. Sometimes he wakes up in the night with leg pain, and when he does, he finishes the night in his recliner chair. Keeping his leg in the dependent position at night seems to help the pain go away.

On physical assessment, you find a round ulcer measuring approximately 3.0 centimeters in circumference located slightly above the left lateral malleolus. The ulcer, although shallow, is a full-thickness wound. The wound bed is pale pink, edges are even with yellow fibrin clinging to the edges, no necrosis, and minimal serous exudate on the dressing that had been applied the day before. There is no odor or surrounding erythema. The dorsalis pedis and posterior tibialis are not palpable. The leg and foot, which have been in a dependent position for several hours, have a purple red color. The color changes to a pale pink when Sam raises his leg above his heart for a few minutes. When direct pressure is applied to the nail beds, the capillary refill takes longer than 3 seconds.

An ABI, done in the home, is 0.5. The complete wound assessment, including the ABI, is communicated to the primary care physician along with the recommendation for a vascular consult. The topical treatment that is selected is one that provides moist wound healing and is not indicated for heavily exudating wounds. A hydrogel or hydrocolloid are two possible options. Wound cleansing can include either normal saline or a wound cleanser. Should normal saline be the choice for cleansing, the psi of the delivery system must be considered. (Refer to Chapter 4, Basics of Wound Management, for cleansing information.) A hydrogel impregnated gauze is selected, and it is held in place with a Kerlix dressing. Sam's wife is instructed in wound care while Sam awaits his physician appointment. They are both instructed about the signs and symptoms of complications and when to call the physician.

Sam is a candidate for revascularization, which he promptly has. Following surgery, ulcer care is selected to provide moist wound healing. The ulcer will heal quickly due to the increase in blood to the leg and foot. Dietary instruction includes a diabetic diet with a focus on low fat. A light exercise program of walking is also included in his rehabilitation to assist with weight control and build any needed collateral circulation in his left leg. Sam is instructed not to use any compression or support stockings in the future due to his atherosclerosis.

Note: Although this was carried out in the home as part of the assessment for a baseline, the reliability of an ABI can be questioned and can give a falsely high reading since Sam is a recently diagnosed non–insulin-dependent diabetic. Due to the vessel disease that can be present in a diabetic, most consider an ABI to be inconclusive, requiring more sophisticated studies to determine blood flow.

REFERENCES

Bickley, L. S., and Hockelman, R. A. 1999. *Bates' guide to physical examination and history taking*, 7th ed. Philadelphia: Lippincott.

Doughty, D. B., Waldrop, J., and Ramunds, J. 2000. Lower-extremity ulcers of vascular etiology. In R. A. Bryant (Ed.) *Acute and chronic wounds: Nursing management* (2d ed.) (265–300). St. Louis, MO: Mosby.

Falanga, V. 1997. Venous ulceration: Assessment, classification, and management. In *Chronic wound care: A clinical source book for healthcare professionals,* 2d ed., eds. D. Krasner and D. Kane, 169–170. Wayne, PA: Health Management Publications.

Holloway, G. A. 1997. Arterial ulcers: Assessment, classification, and management. In *Chronic wound care: A clinical source book for healthcare professionals,* 2d ed., eds. D. Krasner and D. Kane, 158–172. Wayne, PA: Health Management Publications.

Morison, M. et al. 1997. *Nursing management of chronic wounds,* 2d ed. Philadelphia: Mosby, 198–199.

Rubano, J. J., and Kerstein, M. D. 1998. Arterial insufficiency and vasculitides. *Journal of Wound, Ostomy and Continence Nursing* 25 (3), 147–157.

Salcrido, R. C. (Ed.) 2001. Arterial vs. venous ulcers: Diagnosis and treatments. *Skin and Wound Care* 14(3), 146.

Siegel, A. 1998. Noninvasive vascular testing. In *Wound care: A collaborative practice manual for physical therapists and nurses,* eds. C. Sussman and B. M. Bates-Jensen, 127–135. Gaithersburg, MD: Aspen Publishers, Inc.

Sieggreen, M. Y., and Kline, R. A. 2000. Vascular ulcers. In S. Baranoski & E. A. Ayello (Eds.), *Wound care essentials: Practice principles* (271–310) Philadelphia, PA: Lippincott Williams & Wilkins.

Steed, D. 1997. Diabetic wounds: Assessment, classification and management. In *Chronic wound care: A clinical source book for healthcare professionals,* 2d ed., eds. D. Krasner and D. Kane, 173–174. Wayne, PA: Health Management Publications.

Wound, Ostomy and Continence Nurses Society. 2002. Guidelines for management of wounds in patients with lower-extremity arterial disease. Glenview, IL: Author.

Patient Guide: Guidelines for Patients with Peripheral Arterial Disease

WHAT IS PERIPHERAL ARTERIAL DISEASE?

Your circulatory system is made up of the heart, arteries, veins and capillaries. The flow of blood through your body, which is needed to provide nourishment and oxygen to your cells, is your "circulation."

Your arteries carry oxygen-rich blood to all parts of you body. Normally, the blood flows easily through the arteries. In arterial disease, the arteries become narrowed or blocked, and the vessels cannot carry enough blood to the legs and feet.

If the blockage develops slowly, smaller arteries will develop over time and allow some blood to flow around the narrowed area. This is called "collateral circulation."

WHAT ARE THE SIGNS AND SYMPTOMS OF ARTERIAL DISEASE?

Signs and symptoms of decreased blood flow will involve changes in the way your legs and feet look and feel. You may experience:

- pain when walking
- pain at rest
- decrease in leg hair growth
- pallor (or paleness) of leg or foot when raised
- blue/red coloring of the foot
- numbness or tingling
- cool temperature of the skin
- sore or wound that will not heal

WHO IS AT RISK FOR DEVELOPING ARTERIAL DISEASE?

The more risk factors a person has, the more likely he or she will develop arterial disease. The risk factors for arterial disease include:

- smoking
- high blood pressure
- heart disease
- family history of arterial disease
- stress
- high cholesterol
- diabetes
- overweight
- age

HOW CAN ARTERIAL DISEASE BE CONTROLLED OR PREVENTED?

Arterial disease (atherosclerosis) cannot totally be cured or prevented, but you can control certain risk factors by changing you health habits.

Smoking

Tobacco in any form should be avoided. Nicotine causes the blood vessels to constrict, which prevents the normal amount of blood from reaching the organs and extremities and increase the risk of atherosclerosis. Smoking also decreases the amount of oxygen in the blood and may be associated with blood clot formation.

Diet

By reducing cholesterol and saturated fats in the diet, you may reduce the risk of atherosclerosis.

High Blood Pressure

Untreated high blood pressure (hypertension) adds to the workload of the heart and creates stress on the arteries. Have your blood pressure checked regularly and take medications as ordered by your physician. Your physician may suggest stress management classes or a self-restricted diet.

Diabetes

People with diabetes are especially prone to atherosclerosis. It is important to follow the recommendations of a health care team regarding diet, treatment, and medications.

Exercise

Mild, regular, or daily exercise aids in the control of atherosclerosis.

FOOT CARE

When blood flow to the legs is decreased, small injuries to the feet or toes may result in serious infections, sores, or tissue death (gangrene). You need to:

- AVOID situations that might cause a foot injury.
- NEVER expose your feet to extreme heat or cold or to strong chemicals.
- WASH and dry your feet thoroughly, but do not soak.
- AVOID going barefoot.
- WEAR new shoes only for short periods of time.
- INSPECT your shoes. Check inside your shoes for any objects that could injure your feet.

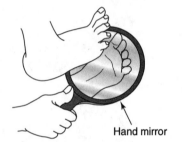
Hand mirror

- INSPECT your feet daily. This is especially important if you have diabetes and/or decreased sensation in your feet.
- USE a mirror if you have trouble seeing your feet. Ask someone to help you.
- CHECK for areas of redness, warmth, swelling, sores, or drainage.
- KEEP your feet clean and dry. Use a moisturizer daily.
- CUT toenails straight across and no shorter than the length of the toe. Round corners with a fine emery board.
- CORNS, calluses, and bunions should be treated by a physician or nurse.
- SPECIAL SHOES or inserts may reduce callus formation and promote control.

CONCLUSION

With recent advances in vascular surgery, atherosclerosis may be treated with a low risk of complications. Surgery may improve or remove symptoms and restore you to a more independent lifestyle. Surgery does not cure atherosclerosis. The disease process is still present. You can help to control this. A firm commitment to keep follow-up appointments with your physician and reduce risk factors will help to control further disease.

CHAPTER 8

Venous Stasis Ulcers

Julie Phelps Maloy

Venous stasis ulcers are the most common type of lower leg ulcer and are a symptom of underlying venous disease (Figures 8–1, 8–2, 8–3; Color Plates 16, 17, 18). Many are long-standing with duration of over a year, causing embarrassment and anxiety for the patient. Recurrence is common. Some studies have indicated that many of those with a venous ulcer have had their first ulceration before the age of 65 (Falanga 1997, 165). A common complaint of the person with venous insufficiency is swelling, discomfort, and heaviness of their legs. Trauma is frequently reported as the initial cause of the ulceration. Typically, these ulcers are not painful; however, when mild discomfort is present, it is usually relieved by leg elevation. Severe, unrelieved pain is suggestive of a different etiology. It is not uncommon for the patient with a venous stasis ulcer to have a history of deep vein thrombosis or previous surgery for varicose veins. Treatment and preventative measures focus on improving venous blood flow and removing the impediments to wound healing. These goals cannot be successfully achieved without the understanding and cooperation of the patient.

ETIOLOGY

Normal Anatomy of the Venous System

Deep Veins

- carry blood under pressure back to the heart
- contain valves to prevent backflow of blood
- are located within the fascia

Superficial Veins

- carry blood under low pressure

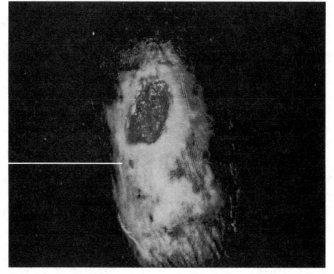

healed closed area

Figure 8–1 Full-Thickness Venous Stasis Ulcer on Dark-Skinned Person. Healed skin will remain light.

Clinical Objectives:
(1) Clean
(2) Keep moist
(3) Manage exudate
(4) Manage edema
See Color Plate 16.

- contain valves to prevent backflow of blood
- drain into deeper veins
- are located outside of the fascia

Perforating Veins

- connect the deep and superficial veins
- contain valves to prevent backflow into superficial veins

Mechanisms of Venous Return

- calf muscle contraction (walking, etc.)
- variations in intra-abdominal and intrathoracic pressure
- venous valves, which allow unidirectional blood blow from superficial veins to deep veins

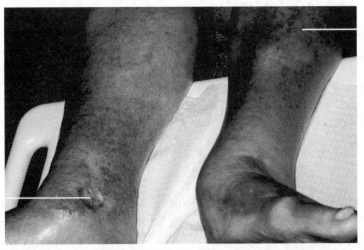

healed ulcer

ulcer, slough base

Figure 8–2 Venus Stasis Ulcer, Right Medial Ankle. Note edema, gaiter staining, and closed wound on left leg.

Clinical Objectives:
(1) Clean
(2) Keep moist
(3) Manage exudate
(4) Manage edema
See Color Plate 17.

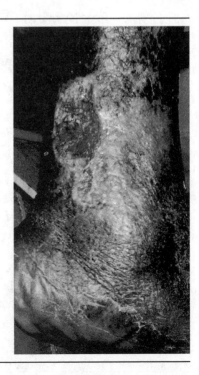

Figure 8–3 Venous Stasis Ulcer. Shallow wound bed, irregular shape, wound bed ruddy red with some yellow slough.

Clinical Objectives:
(1) Clean
(2) Keep moist
(3) Manage exudate
(4) Manage edema
See Color Plate 18.

Venous Stasis Ulcers

A cascade of events occurs with venous disease, including increased hydrostatic pressure, venous hypertension, and venous stasis ulceration. In chronic venous hypertension, damaged valves in the deep and perforating veins with backflow to superficial veins cause:

- dilation of veins
- edema
- increased pressure in the superficial veins
- further valve damage

Various theories as to the exact cause of the ulcerations are debated and include:

- the Fibrin Cuff Theory (Falanga 1997, 166; Morison and Moffatt 1997, 183)
- the White Cell Trapping Theory (Morison and Moffatt 1997, 183)
- the Mechanical Theory (Falanga 1997, 166–168; Morison and Moffatt 1997, 183)

ASSESSMENT

Predisposing Factors

- family history
- gender (higher incidence in women)
- pregnancy
- low-fiber diet
- obesity
- leg injury
- occupations that require standing
- smoking
- history of major leg trauma
- history of deep vein thrombosis (DVT)
- history of venous ligation or stripping

Clinical Signs

See Appendix A and Appendix B for a comparison of venous insufficiency, arterial insufficiency, and peripheral neuropathy.

- brown/red staining of the skin in the gaiter area (hemosiderin staining)
- extremely dry, scaly skin or weepy, itchy, and erythematous skin (stasis eczema, dermatitis)
- peripheral edema that increases with prolonged standing and/or sitting (Prolonged edema gives the leg the appearance of an upside-down champagne bottle.)
- distention of tiny veins on medial aspect of the foot (ankle flare)
- induration of the tissue of lower leg (lipodermatosclerosis)
- thinning of the dermis
- history of an ulcer
- non-pitting ankle edema that doesn't resolve with elevation (woody fibrosis)

Ulcer (Typical Appearance)

- irregularly shaped wound (not typically round or with even wound edges)
- location on the medial aspect of the lower leg and ankle (common)
- painless (Patient may have a dull ache or heavy feeling particularly at night; unrelieved pain indicates further complicating factors.)
- extension into the dermal skin layer (frequent)
- ruddy red wound bed, with granular tissue; may have some yellow slough or yellow to brown fibrin
- exudate present (serous or serosanguineous)
- variable size

The etiology of the ulcer may not be known to patient.

TREATMENT CHOICES

Goals

- reduce edema
- reduce blood pressure in the superficial venous system
- aid venous return to the heart
- utilize appropriate topical therapy to provide moist wound healing
- educate to prevent recurrence

- educate on importance of compression stockings after the ulcer has heeled

Simple Diagnostics

- history and physical assessment
- Doppler ultrasonography: ankle-brachial index (ABI) (Exhibit 7–1, page 142–143)

Further studies could include color-flow duplex imaging to help identify areas of valvular incompetence and/or photoplethysmography.

Compression Wraps (Exhibit 8–1, page 159)

The purpose of compression is to eliminate or reduce edema and to assist with venous return. Controversy exists over the amount of compression.

Effective compression must provide extraluminal pressure greater than intraluminal pressure (Rudolph 1998, 251).

Contraindications include arterial involvement as determined by diagnostics, deep vein thrombosis, cellulitis, severe leg deformity, and acute congestive heart failure.

TIP A lack of wound improvement in two to three weeks is an indication for a complete reassessment of the patient.

Types of Wraps

Follow the manufacturer's instructions. A few examples of different compression wraps are listed below. There are many more available.

- single-layer bandaging (e.g., Unna Boot™, Tubigrip™, Comprilan™)
- multilayer bandaging (e.g., Profore™, Unna-Flex™)
- graduated compression wraps (e.g., Profore™, SurePress™, Duoderm Sustained Compression Bandage™)
- compression wrap systems (e.g., CirAid™, Thera-Boot™, CircPlus™)

Exhibit 8–1 Methods of Edema Management

Elimination and control of edema may be accomplished through leg elevation, exercise, and the use of compression therapy. A combination of the above-mentioned therapies is often necessary to achieve the desired control of edema in the affected limb(s). Clients should be encouraged to elevate their legs as often as possible and in general to avoid any length of time with their legs in a dependent position. Exercise that works the calf muscle pump while the client is using the appropriate compression garment or wrap should be encouraged. Clients may also find that elevation of the foot of the bed is helpful to facilitate leg elevation while sleeping. This is not useful for the client with heart disease, such as congestive heart failure. It is not unusual to find clients requesting a diuretic or water pill to facilitate the removal of the edema. The health care provider is encouraged to see this as an opportunity to provide client education about the futility of diuretics as a primary treatment for edema. Diuretics may be useful as an adjuvant therapy, especially if a sequential compression pump is to be used for the client with compromised cardiac function; however, diuretics are not a long-term solution to edema management. Appropriate for edema management are leg elevation and exercise, elastic wraps, tubular bandages, paste bandages, four-layer bandaging, graduated compression stockings, and intermittent sequential compression devices. A discussion of each follows.

LEG ELEVATION WITH EXERCISE

Leg elevation facilitates the removal of fluid through utilization of gravity to assist venous return. For leg elevation to be successful, the legs must be higher than the heart. Simply placing the feet on a stool is of no benefit. To facilitate leg elevation, the client may find it helpful to place one or two bricks under the foot end of the bed, which elevates the legs higher than the heart during sleep. It is helpful to demonstrate on the exam table or hospital bed by elevating the legs and then reclining on the surface. Clients should be encouraged to exercise the feet and ankles while elevating the legs. Stress that leg elevation can be intermittent and that total bed rest is not recommended. Intermittent leg elevation during the day for 20–30 minutes at a time for a total of at least two hours a day is a reasonable goal.

COMPRESSION THERAPY (ELASTIC AND TUBULAR BANDAGES)

Compression therapy works with exercise to facilitate the movement of excess fluid from the lower extremity. The level of compression needed for edema secondary to venous disease is approximately 40 mm Hg. For the client who is able to walk and work the calf muscles, 40 mm Hg compression is recommended. A client with dependent edema who is unable to work the calf muscles will not tolerate this level of compression and a lower level of compression (Class 1 or Class 2) should be considered. (See Table 8–1, page 163.) Elastic bandages are relatively easy to apply, inexpensive, and easily removed. As with all compression garments/devices, it is best to apply the bandages within 20 minutes of waking and placing the feet below the level of the heart. Most compression wraps giving at least Class 2 compression are removed at night. Bandages do require practice to apply correctly and the skill needs to be taught to the client and caregiver. Manufacturer's guidelines should always be followed when applying the elastic bandage. The most common application technique is the spiral. Several types of bandages are now available with printed rectangles that when stretched to squares apply the correct level of compression. These markings facilitate correct wrapping of an extremity.

continues

Exhibit 8–1 continued

Tubular bandages provide light compression. One should be careful to select bandages that are tapered at the ankle. Straight tubular bandages provide compression that is higher at the calf than at the ankle. These are not as useful for the client with edema.

PASTE (UNNA BOOT) BANDAGES

Paste bandages such as the Unna Boot are widely used in the treatment of leg ulcers and in the control of edema. The boot was developed in the 1880s by a German physician, Paul Gerson Unna, and consists of a fine gauze impregnated with zinc oxide, gelatin, and glycerin (some varieties also include calamine). The gauze is applied without tension in a circular fashion from the foot to just below the knee. Paste bandages do not provide compression; however, as the boot dries and stiffens, the leg cannot continue to swell. Application of a compression wrap over the boot will enhance compression and protect the client's clothing from the moist paste of the boot. A paste bandage is routinely changed every four to seven days.

FOUR-LAYER BANDAGING

An alternative to the paste bandage is the four-layer bandage developed at Charing Cross Hospital in London. The four-layer bandage provides graduated, sustained compression through the application of a series of layers, providing protection, padding, and compression. The dressing is removed weekly.

GRADUATED COMPRESSION STOCKINGS

Graduated compression stockings assist venous return, thereby reducing edema. The client should be measured and fitted for compression stockings when the edema is absent or minimal. These stockings are then applied before the client has gotten out of bed or at least within 20 minutes of rising. Stockings may be difficult to get on and devices are available to assist in donning. A nonambulatory client does not need moderate or high compression and will likely better tolerate a lower-compression (18–24 mm Hg) stocking. Stockings do wear out and need to be replaced at the frequency recommended by the manufacturer. Many clients prefer to order two stockings (or two pairs) to prolong the life of the individual stocking and allow for laundering.

SEQUENTIAL COMPRESSION THERAPY

Sequential compression therapy has gained popularity for the management of lower extremity edema. The leg sleeve (either knee-high or thigh-high) is divided into 3-,5-, and 10-chamber styles with peak pressures of 45 to 60 mm Hg at the ankle. The sleeve inflates first at the ankle, followed 2.5 seconds later at the calf chambers, and 3 seconds later at the thigh chambers. Each successive chamber inflates less and the total inflation is sustained for approximately 5 seconds followed by complete deflation. The cycle repeats every 7–8 seconds for the prescribed treatment period, which may range from one to two hours twice per day. Clients should be encouraged to follow treatment with application of either a fitted stocking or a compression bandage to maintain edema control. Use of compression therapy at night while sleeping is not recommended. Clients with congestive heart disease should be monitored closely for tolerance of the intravascular fluid burden with compression therapy.

- mechanical graduated or sequential (lymphedema) pumps (e.g., Flow-press, Sof-Pres) Be sure to check the access in your area and the reimbursement of the pumps for the diagnosis of venous stasis ulcers.
  - Treatment is usually performed one to two times per day for specific amount of time.
  - Pumps can be contraindicated for patients with congestive heart failure.

Local Wound Treatment

- Clean the wound with normal saline or a commercially prepared wound cleanser.
- Some compression wraps are impregnated with zinc oxide, gelatin, and glycerin pastes.
- For highly exudating ulcers, use foams, alginates, and hydrofiber dressings under the compression wrap.
- Use hydrocolloid dressings under compression wraps when the wound is no longer highly exudative.
- Moisturize the leg and foot before applying compression.
- Measure the circumference of the leg to document the change in edema. Some measure 2, 6, and 8 inches above the ankle. This provides specific information on the effectiveness of a graduated compression wrap on the edema.
- Compression wraps are not all applied the same way. Some manufacturers recommend a spiral wrap while others recommend a figure eight. Follow the manufacturer's recommendations for the product you have selected to use. It is also wise to be taught how to wrap before attempting to apply a compression wrap to a patient.
- Should leg elevation be used, the leg should be elevated above the level of the heart to be effective.

TIPS • Change the first one or two compression wraps more frequently than the manufacturer of the compression wrap recommends. If the manufacturer suggests weekly changes, change it twice a week for the first one or two changes to assess patient's tolerance to compression and the amount of wound exudate. The amount of exudate will drive your decision on the addition of an absorbent dressing under the compression such as a foam or alginate.
- Cleansing usually removes the odor that is present when the compression wrap is changed.

- Always provide the patient with the signs and symptoms of complications, and what to do should they occur. Look for signs such as:
  - change in appearance of the toes—dusky or purple discoloration
  - increase in amount of discomfort or pain in the extremity
- Should either of the above occur, the patient should call the emergency number that you have provided for your agency and/or remove the compression wrap. Once the edema begins to subside, many patients feel more comfortable with the wrap in place.
- Manage exudate with local wound treatment to prevent periwound maceration.
- Compress until the wound has healed to provide compliance and continuity.

EXPECTED OUTCOMES

- With compression, the wound will decrease dimensions quickly, sometimes with each dressing change.
- Without compression, long-term chronic wound management may be necessary due to the underlying pathology.

PREVENTION

Patient Education

- Explain the cause of ulcerations. Use a simple explanation of the difficulty the blood has in the return to the heart, including the function of support stockings/hosiery.
- Emphasize the importance of the long-term use of support stockings/ compression hosiery (Table 8–1, page 163).
- Tell the patient to elevate legs above the level of the heart when sitting (Exhibit 8–2, page 163).
- Tell the patient to avoid crossing legs.
- Stress exercise.
- Stress weight loss. A restriction of sodium intake is frequently beneficial.
- Counsel on smoking cessation.

See Exhibit 8–3, page 165.

Table 8-1 Vascular Support Options

Level of Support	Examples	Recommendations for Use
Light support (8–14 mm Hg)	Fashion hosiery Jobst Sigvarus	Edema prevention for persons engaged in activities/work that require standing/sitting without much activity; examples: beautician, cashier, factory worker, some nursing positions
Antiembolism stockings (16–18 mm Hg)	Anti-EM/GP (Jobst) TED stockings	Deep vein thrombosis prophylaxis Nonambulatory clients with edema
Low compression (18–24 mm Hg)	Relief (Jobst) Elastic wraps Paste bandage	Nonambulatory clients with edema Nonambulatory clients with edema failing 16–18 mm Hg stockings Clients with dependent edema
Low to moderate compression (25–35 mm Hg)	Fast-Fit (Jobst) Custom fit Double reverse elastic wrap Four-layer bandage	Edema secondary to venous insufficiency Edema in client able to participate in exercise rehab
Moderate compression (30–40 mm Hg)	Ultimate (Jobst) Custom stocking (Jobst, Sigvarus) Sequential pump Four-layer bandage (Profore, SurePress)	Edema with/without ulceration Edema that persists in spite of lower-level compression options Ulcer that failed to heal after 6 months
High compression (40–50 mm Hg)	Vairox (Jobst) Custom stockings (Jobst, Sigvarus) Sequential pump	Edema secondary to lymphedema

Note: Check with Medicare and private insurance about reimbursement for support hose.

Exhibit 8–2 Patient Guide: Leg Elevation and Exercise

DEFINITION

Elevation of the legs higher than the level of the heart, with or without foot and ankle exercise, to allow gravity to assist in the removal of fluid from the legs

continues

Exhibit 8–2 continued

ADVANTAGES

- no costs associated with the procedure
- effective when used regularly in combination with other form(s) of compression bandaging or stockings
- no special equipment required
- involves client in active participation in edema reduction

DISADVANTAGES

- Exercise/elevation requires consistent performance in order to be of benefit.
- Some people may be unable to elevate legs higher than the heart (e.g., clients with obesity, congestive heart failure, or orthopedic limitations).
- Sitting may not be allowed at work for leg elevation.
- Exercise/elevation may be ineffective in some forms of swelling.

EQUIPMENT NEEDED

- clean surface upon which to recline
- minute timer (optional)

FREQUENCY

Every two–three hours during the day for 20–30 minutes for a total of two or more hours per day

WHEN TO USE

When edema of the lower extremities occurs due to impaired venous return

WHEN *NOT* TO USE

- if you are very obese
- if you have hardening of the arteries (atherosclerosis) and pain with leg elevation
- if you have congestive heart failure and a limited ability to recline in a horizontal position
- if you have other medical conditions that limit your ability to recline in a horizontal position

continues

Exhibit 8–2 continued

PROCEDURE

1. Recline horizontally on a clean, comfortable surface (bed or recliner chair).

2. Elevate legs approximately 30 degrees so that feet are higher than the heart. Rest feet against wall or footboard of bed.

3. Set timer for 20 to 30 minutes (optional).

4. With one leg at a time, flex and extend foot against wall or footboard, then make circles (rotate) with the foot/ankle. Do 5–10 repetitions with each foot, then rest and repeat until timer goes off.

5. Remove and rewrap leg if compression bandage is being used.

EXPECTED RESULTS

Your swelling and pain/discomfort are relieved with leg elevation.

HELPFUL HINTS

- Use of a kitchen-type minute timer is helpful to ensure an adequate amount of time.

- Work up to 20–30 minutes gradually if it is too much when starting out.

- Be creative at work in looking for opportunities to exercise (walking, stair climbing, marching in place).

Exhibit 8–3 Patient Guide: Guidelines for Patients with Venous Insufficiency or Wounds

GIVE YOUR LEGS A REST

- Elevate your feet above your heart while sleeping and at regular times during the day (elevate foot of bed or mattress).

- Avoid work that requires you to stand or sit with your feet on the ground for long periods. Change positions frequently.

- Take walks to help leg muscles "pump" fluids into your legs.

GIVE YOUR LEGS SUPPORT

- Wear professionally made support stockings that apply pressure from ankle to knee or other compression devices. (Your physician can help you choose the kind that is right for you and send you to a professional who will properly measure your legs for stocking size.)

continues

Exhibit 8–3 continued

- Have at least two pairs of support stockings available so you can change them daily. After laundering, hang them up to dry. Do not put them in a dryer.

- Always put on support stockings early in the morning before fluid pools in lower legs.

- Wear support stockings all day and then remove them in the evening when going to sleep.

- Buy new stockings every six months so their strength doesn't wear out.

- Avoid ACE® bandages. It is extremely difficult to wrap them properly to provide the pressure you need.

- If your physician has prescribed the use of a compression pump, follow the instructions completely. It may take a little time to adjust to the pumping procedure.

TAKE CARE OF YOUR SKIN

- Wash your lower legs and feet regularly with mild soap and water.

- Use moisturizing creams and emollients after washing. Don't put lotion on the wounds. It is important not to use petroleum or lanolin-based creams when wearing stockings that contain latex. Your physician or pharmacist may suggest appropriate brands.

- Be particularly careful to avoid activities that are likely to cause injury to legs or feet. *Prevention is very important.*

WATCH FOR SKIN CHANGES

Pay particular attention to signs of progressive venous insufficiency:

- **swelling** that does not go away quickly when you lie down

- **discoloration,** especially brownish skin discoloration around ankles and lower legs

- **dryness and/or itching** in the same areas

- **any wound or bruise** that doesn't go away within a week

IF YOU HAVE A WOUND

- Keep it clean. Keep minor wounds clean and protect with a bandage.

- Avoid strong antiseptics. Many antiseptics such as hydrogen peroxide, povidone–iodine, and sodium hypochlorite can damage skin and interfere with healing.

- Always wear support stockings during your daily activities. If it is difficult to wear them over the bandage, put on a knee-length nylon stocking first and wear the support stocking over it.

continues

Exhibit 8–3 continued

- Watch the wound carefully. You will need to describe any changes to your physician. Remember that any wound may turn into a chronic wound, and early treatment has been shown to be beneficial.

IF YOUR WOUND DOESN'T HEAL IN ONE WEEK

Don't put off seeing your physician. *Any wound that doesn't heal in a week should be seen by your physician.*

REMEMBER

- You are a vital part of your treatment program and it is essential that you faithfully follow all medical directions.

- Always consult your health care professional before making any change to your health care routine, if you have questions, or if your symptoms are becoming worse.

CASE STUDY

Mrs. Jan Evens, 66 years old, lives with her husband in a one-story home in a small Midwestern community. She has three adult children living nearby. Jan weighs 170 pounds and is 5 feet 5 inches tall. She has been a smoker, although she hasn't smoked in the last 10 years and has recently retired from a packaging company where she worked, for the past 15 years, standing on an assembly line. Jan is not a diabetic.

Jan has been admitted to home care following surgery for a ruptured diverticular abscess and a colostomy. She has an open abdominal incision requiring a skilled nurse visit and has a long-standing lower leg ulcer. The physician's orders for the skilled nursing visit included not only care of the abdominal incision and colostomy teaching, but also ulcer care. Jan told her home care nurse she has had the ulcer for several years, and it has always embarrassed her. She usually wore slacks to hide it even during the summer. In the past, Jan treated the ulcer with various creams and antibiotic ointments and a bandage. It would get smaller, but it never healed completely.

An assessment of her lower leg reveals a moderate amount of edema of her lower leg and foot. Jan states that she had noticed that if she elevated her leg at night when she watched television, the swelling decreased. She does not have any leg pain. There is red/brown discoloration of the skin above her ankle (hemosiderin staining), prominent superficial leg veins, distention of the veins on the medial aspect of the foot (ankle flare), a hardened, indurated texture to the skin (lipodermatosclerosis), and dry, flaky skin (stasis dermatitis). The ulcer is a full-thickness wound on the medial aspect of the lower leg, measuring 6.0 cm long by 4.0 cm wide and approximately 1.0 cm deep. The wound edges are irregular and have a white discoloration (maceration from wound exudate). The wound bed is approximately 75 percent red, granular tissue and 25 percent yellow, fibrinous slough. The gauze dressing, applied the day before, is saturated with tannish colored drainage. The wound has no odor. An ABI, done in the home, is 0.8. A full report of the assessment findings including the ABI was telephoned to the physician.

A foam dressing was chosen to cover the wound. A hydrocolloid, alginate, or hydrofiber would also be appropriate; however, in this case, a foam was chosen to absorb the wound exudate evidenced by the maceration at the wound edges. In addition, a compression wrap was applied after obtaining a measurement of the leg circumference 2, 6, and 10 inches above the ankle. The measurements provided a reference point for the expected decrease in the edema with the use of compression. The first wrap was changed in four days to assess the wound and the patient's tolerance of compression. The patient was instructed to call if there was pain or blue/purple discoloration of the toes. Jan tolerated compression well and the foam dressing adequately absorbed the wound exudate. The compression wrap was changed weekly thereafter. The wound was completely healed in less than six months. The patient wore light compression hosiery after healing. Light compression was selected to reduce recurrence and increase compliance. Dietary instructions, including methods to increase fiber and lower weight, were given to Jan. A light exercise program of walking was initiated to help with weight control and to increase the pumping action of the calf muscle, thereby assisting with venous return to the heart. Understanding the underlying cause of the ulceration, weight loss, regular exercise, and light compression were key elements in a prevention program for Jan.

REFERENCES

Falanga, V. 1997. Venous ulceration: Assessment, classification and management. In *Chronic wound care: A clinical source book for healthcare professionals*, 2d ed., eds. D. Krasner and D. Kane. Wayne, PA: Health Management Publications, 165–171.

Kunimoto, B. T. 2001. Management and prevention of venous leg ulcers: A literature-guided approach. *Ostomy Wound Management*, 47(6), 36–49.

Kunimoto, B. T., Casling, M., Gulliner, W., Houghton, P. Orstead, H., and Sibbold, R. G. 2001. Best practice for prevention and treatment of venous leg ulcers. *Ostomy Wound Management*, 47(2), 34–50.

Morison, M., and Moffatt, C. 1997. Leg ulcers. In *Nursing management of chronic wounds*, 2d ed., eds. M. Morison et al. Philadelphia: Mosby, 177–220.

Rudolph, D. 1998. Pathophysiology and management of venous ulcers. *Journal of Wound, Ostomy, and Continence Nursing*, 25(5), 248–255.

Sieggreen, M. Y., and Kline, R. A. 2000. Vascular ulcers. In S. Baranoski and E. A. Ayello (eds.) *Wound care essentials: Practice principles* (271–310). Philadelphia, PA: Lippincott Williams & Wilkins.

BIBLIOGRAPHY

Siegel, A. 1998. Noninvasive vascular testing. In *Wound care: A collaborative practice manual for physical therapists and nurses*, eds. C. Sussman and B. M. Bates-Jensen. Gaithersburg, MD: Aspen Publishers, Inc., 127–135.

CHAPTER 9

Lower Leg Ulcers with Mixed Disease

Julie Phelps Maloy

It is not uncommon to be asked to evaluate and recommend treatment for an ulcer on the lower leg that clinically resembles a venous stasis ulcer but, after a complete assessment, is also shown to have arterial involvement (Figure 9–1; Color Plate 19). This patient has mixed disease or venous stasis disease with underlying arterial involvement. This means not only are there incompetent valves in the veins creating difficulty with the venous return, but also probable atherosclerosis in the arteries restricting the blood flow into the extremity. The patient may or may not also be a diabetic. Compression is the treatment of choice for venous stasis ulcers (Chapter 8), however, only if there is adequate blood supply to the extremity evidenced by vascular studies. If you jump to a conclusion that the ulcer is a venous stasis ulcer based on a visual assessment, you could compress a patient who is not a candidate for compression, further restricting the blood flow to the extremity and hastening an amputation. Some have estimated that as many as 21 percent of patients with lower leg ulcers have an arterial component (Morison & Moffatt 1997, 186). It is extremely important to know the etiology of the ulcers for which you recommend treatments.

ETIOLOGY

Chronic venous stasis ulcers are caused by damaged valves in the deep and perforating veins, with backflow to superficial veins causing:

- dilation of veins
- edema
- increased pressure in the superficial veins
- further valve damage

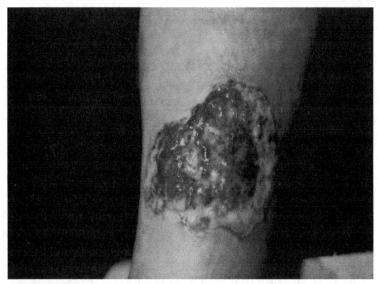

Figure 9–1 Ulcer with Mixed Disease. Patient is not a surgical candidate.
Clinical Objectives:
(1) Prevent infection
(2) Provide protection
(3) Absorb exudate
See Color Plate 19.

Arterial ulcers (refer to Chapter 7, Arterial Ulcers) are caused by a lack of blood supply with the most common cause being atherosclerosis.

ASSESSMENT

Risk Factors

- hypertension
- smoking
- diabetes
- hyperlipidemia
- obesity
- family history
- occupations requiring standing

Clinical Signs

Lower Leg

- brown staining of the skin (hemosiderin staining)
- dry, scaly skin (stasis eczema)
- peripheral edema (can be only slight)
- thinning of the dermis
- induration of the tissue of the lower leg (lipodermatosclerosis)
- distention of the tiny veins on the medial aspect of the foot (ankle flare)
- pulses palpable or not palpable in the dorsalis pedis and posterior tibialis
- possible accompanying cellulitis
- possible thickened, yellow, fragile toenails

Ulcer

- irregularly shaped or rounded wound edges
- located on the medial, front, or lateral aspect of the lower leg or ankle
- pain, cramping, or burning (can be masked if the patient is a diabetic)
- pale or ruddy and granular wound bed
- exudate (usually present)
- etiology due to trauma or unknown by the patient
- long-standing duration
- slough or dry eschar in the wound bed

Complications

- wound infection
- gangrene (black or brown necrotic tissue caused by a lack of blood supply, frequently at the most distal aspects of the leg and foot; if toe is affected, can wither into a hard mass and separate by autolysis)
- amputation

TREATMENT CHOICES

Goals

Goals are dependent upon the physical condition of the patient.

- Establish adequate circulation to the affected area when the patient is a surgical candidate (Arterial Ulcers, Chapter 7).
- After establishing adequate circulation surgically,
  - Reduce the edema.
  - Utilize appropriate topical therapy.
- For the nonsurgical candidate,
  - Utilize appropriate topical therapy.
  - Do not include compression therapy. Compression therapy further restricts the compromised arterial blood flow to the leg.

Diagnostics

- history and physical assessment
- noninvasive studies of the arterial system using a Doppler ultrasound to determine the ankle-brachial index (ABI) (Exhibit 7–1, page 142)
  - A normal ABI is considered to be 0.9–1.1.
  - Claudication can occur between 0.5 and 0.6.
  - Tissue loss and rest pain (signaling a threatened limb) can occur at < 0.5.

  Most consider an ABI to be invalid in a diabetic patient. The increased atherosclerosis with resulting calcified vessels causes a falsely elevated ABI.
- further vascular evaluation

Surgical Intervention for Revascularization

See bibliography for resources containing further surgical information.

Medical Management

Nonsurgical candidates require good wound care and patient education. Nurses need to be aware that without restoring an adequate blood supply, this is usually a nonhealing wound that can get progressively worse.

TIP Even though this ulcer can strongly resemble a venous stasis ulcer, don't treat it using compression if an ABI indicates this is a threatened limb. Compression is not an option for all patients with lower leg ulcers and edema.

Local Wound Management

- Clean the wound with normal saline or a commercially prepared wound cleanser.
- Utilize wound dressings that provide a moist wound environment, preventing the wound from drying out. A dry wound causes increased cell death and necrosis. *Note:* The current thought is that heels and toes are an exception to the moist wound dressings rule: If heels and toes are covered with hard, black eschar, leave them covered with the black eschar unless there are signs and symptoms of infection, leakage of exudate, or odor. Removing eschar that has no other symptoms increases the opportunity for infection and can quickly lead to an amputation due to the already compromised blood supply to the area.
- Select a dressing that meets the needs of the wound (see Chapter 5, Wound Treatments).

PREVENTION

Patient Education

- Explain the underlying cause of the ulceration(s).
- Discuss blood glucose control with the diabetic patient.
- Counsel on cessation of smoking.
- Stress weight control and a mild exercise program, both for weight control and to build collateral circulation if the patient is able to tolerate this without intermittent claudication. Explain the benefits of a low-fat diet.
- Discuss blood pressure management (including stress reduction classes, if appropriate).
- Include pharmacologic education of drug interactions and reactions for patients on medication.
- Explain signs and symptoms of complications along with what to do should they occur:
  - Look for deepening of the ulcer along with increasing amounts of exudate, erythema, streaks of red running up the leg, pain, and/or the presence of black tissue (eschar or gangrene).
  - Call the physician, or if an emergent situation go to the emergency department.

CASE STUDY

Randy Rudicle was referred to your agency following discharge from the hospital. He had been admitted to the hospital because his recently diagnosed diabetes mellitus was poorly controlled. His medical history includes coronary heart disease and diabetes, which he had attempted to control by dietary measures. He had angioplasty with stent placement in two coronary arteries six months earlier. He required home care follow-up for his recently diagnosed diabetes mellitus, which now requires the use of insulin. He also requires a skilled nurse for treatment of a long-standing ulcer on his right lower leg. Randy is 66 years old, 6 feet tall, and 270 pounds. He has been a two-pack-a-day cigarette smoker, although he had stopped smoking six months ago when his coronary artery disease was diagnosed. He is retired; however, he had worked in an industrial environment on an assembly line most of his working years. In addition to his other medical conditions, Randy has an ulcer on the front of his lower right leg. He fell down a few steps of a ladder when he was painting the trim on his house and skinned the front of his leg a year ago. He has tried several home remedies and, to his frustration, the ulcer has increased in size. Randy's leg has a small amount of edema, which is unilateral. The right lower leg has some hemosiderin staining extending beyond the ulcer approximately 4.0 cm. There is not any induration. The gauze 4 × 4 dressing, which was applied in the early am, is saturated with tan drainage. There is no odor. The ulcer, measuring 5.0 cm long by 3.0 cm wide, is oval in shape with even wound edges. The wound bed has a ruddy granular appearance. The ulcer is now a full-thickness ulcer. The ulcer has many of the clinical signs of a venous stasis ulcer; however, due to Randy's diagnosis of diabetes, an ABI is not a reliable test to determine arterial involvement. A referral from the physician for a vascular evaluation at a vascular laboratory will be necessary before a complete treatment plan for the wound can be identified. The testing reveals arterial involvement requiring revascularization. Randy does not want any further surgical procedures at this time. He is overwhelmed with all of his recent medical problems. His choice is for a more conservative path for wound care.

The care of this patient and the long-term management is complex. It will be necessary to follow up on and reinforce the diabetes education that began in the hospital, including dietary reinforcement, the correct administration of insulin, blood glucose monitoring, proper foot care, and the potential for slow-healing wounds. In addition, any further education on coronary heart disease could be indicated along with providing support for Randy's progress on smoking cessation and stress management. A light exercise program to help with weight control and to decrease stress would be ideal when Randy is no longer homebound; however, with the complication of arterial disease in his extremities, he could experience intermittent claudication from a decrease of oxygen to the muscles (refer to Chapter 7, Arterial Ulcers). It will be necessary for the nurse to educate Randy on good wound care utilizing the principles of moist wound healing. The signs and symptoms of wound complications requiring a call to his physician should also be included. The probability of wound healing is minimal in a wound that has the complication of significant arterial disease. The dressing selection should include one that will provide moist wound healing, absorb the exudate, protect the wound from further trauma, and be manageable and affordable for Randy and his wife. This could include a foam, alginate, hydrofiber, or composite dressing (see Chapter 5, Wound Treatments). Not all wounds have an outcome that nurses have come to expect. Randy's decision could be the best for him at the present. He could have difficulty in healing after revascularization until his diabetes is in better long-term control. Either way, an amputation could occur in his future.

REFERENCE

Morison, M., and Moffatt, C. 1997. Leg ulcers. In *Nursing management of chronic wounds*, 2d ed. eds. M. Morison et al. 177–220. Philadelphia, PA: Mosby.

BIBLIOGRAPHY

O'Brien, S. P. et al. 1998. Epidemiology, risk factors, and management of peripheral vascular disease. *Ostomy/Wound Management* 44(9), 68–75.
Siegel, A. 1998. Noninvasive vascular testing. In *Wound care: A collaborative practice manual for physical therapists and nurses.* eds. C. Sussman and B. M. Bates-Jensen, 127–135. Gaithersburg, MD: Aspen Publishers, Inc.

CHAPTER 10

Diabetic Neuropathic Foot Ulcers

Julie Phelps Maloy

Diabetes is a complicated chronic disease. The information presented here is not meant to oversimplify diabetes. A high blood glucose can contribute to many complications. One set of complications is the diabetic neuropathic foot ulcer. A person with diabetes can have venous stasis or arterial ulcers; however, when the reference is made to a diabetic ulcer, it is most commonly considered to be a neuropathic ulcer located on the plantar surface of the foot. Various authorities report that two-thirds of those with diabetes will have foot pathology by the year 2010. Foot ulcers are the most common cause of hospitalization among those with diabetes. Over one-half of the lower limb amputations are performed on diabetic patients. Eighty-five percent of diabetes-related amputations are preceded by a foot ulcer (Armstrong et al. 1998, 123 and Kravitz et al. 2003, 69). Research has shown that the amputation of one toe is enough to contribute to the development of deformities of the remaining toes and to the formation of a new ulcer on the same foot as well as the other (contralateral) foot (Levin 1998, 129–130). Many factors contribute to the foot ulcer, including lack of sensation; bone and muscle changes resulting in toe, ankle, and foot deformities; lack of perspiration; friction; and callus buildup. Diabetics have impaired wound healing ability. Once the ulceration occurs, the problem is compounded. If the wound is not aggressively treated, infection quickly occurs, leading to gangrene and an amputation. This sets the stage for further amputations, and the cycle continues.

ETIOLOGY

Many factors contribute to diabetic neuropathic foot ulcers. These factors usually includes sensory, motor, and autonomic neuropathy. These conditions are not reversible and will continue to worsen over time.

Background

An increased blood glucose interferes with the structural integrity of collagen, enzymatic reactions, and the functions of the cell membrane. (More in-depth information on diabetes and wound healing is found in Levin et al. 1993, Mulder 2000, and Steed 1997, 172–177.)

Peripheral Neuropathy

Motor

- toe changes (claw toes/hammer toes)
- thinning of the fat pad over the ball of the foot (metatarsal head)
- atrophy of the muscles (interosseous) of the metatarsals

Sensory

- loss of sensation

Autonomic Neuropathy

- increased blood flow leads to increased bone reabsorption, which can cause joint collapse and Charcot foot
- decreased perspiration leads to dry, cracked skin

Peripheral Vascular Disease

- impaired wound healing
- artherosclerosis (occurs at a younger age and advances more rapidly in the person with diabetes)
- cholesterol emboli

Summary

- Lower leg has shiny skin, dependent rubor, hair loss, subcutaneous fat atrophy, and delayed superficial plexus filling time.
- Atherosclerosis of the vessels in the leg leads to a decrease in blood flow to the leg and foot and therefore a decrease of oxygen and nutrition to the extremity.
- A decrease in touch sensation, temperature sensation, and pain perception creates an inability to feel any discomfort with the shoes or any trauma to the feet.

- A lack of perspiration creates dry feet that crack, providing a hiding place for bacteria and a potential for infection.
- Deterioration of the muscles results in changes in the toes, causing a change in the weight distribution through the forefoot.
- Deterioration of the bones in the foot (Charcot foot) leads to deformities and changes in the weight distribution of the foot.
- Sliding of foot causes friction and callus build-up. If a cavity forms under the callus, an ulcer is formed. Dry cracked skin and the bacteria contained there empty bacteria into the ulcer bed, leading to infection, gangrene, and possibly amputation.

CHARCOT FOOT

See Figures 10–1 and 10–2; Color Plate 20.

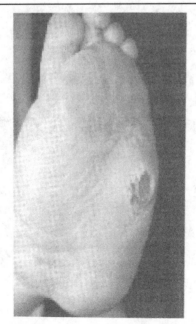

Figure 10–1 Classic Charcot Rocker-Bottom Foot Deformity. Note ulceration over bony deformity surrounded by callus formation.

Stages of Development (Levin 1998, 132)

First Stage (Acute Stage)

- Usually there has been some type of trauma to the foot or ankle.
- The clinical picture is hot, red, swollen, with bounding pulses, resembling a cellulitis.
- Treatment is non–weight bearing, which continues until the skin temperature returns to normal. A total contact case is often used.

Second Stage

- This stage occurs because the patient ambulated in the first stage.
- The foot develops fragmentation (pieces of bone break off) and fractures.
- The toes take on a pointed appearance.
- Changes can develop as early as two to three weeks after stage 1.

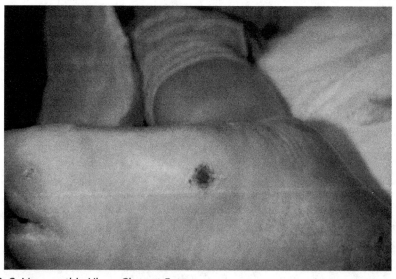

Figure 10–2 Neuropathic Ulcer; Charcot Foot.
Clinical Objectives:
(1) Off-loading techniques
(2) Manage infection if present
(3) Manage exudate
See Color Plate 20.

Third Stage

- The foot is deformed due to the collapse of the joints in stage 2.
- The clinical picture is a rocker-bottom/clubfoot look due to the collapse of the plantar arch.

Fourth Stage

- Should the patient continue to walk on the foot, unprotected ulceration develops due to the shift of pressure.
- Ulceration quickly leads to infection, gangrene, and eventual amputation.

ASSESSMENT

See Appendix A at the end of the book for a comparison of venous insufficiency, arterial insufficiency, and peripheral neuropathy.

Risk Factors (Elftman 1998, 315–345 and Kravitz, McGuire, & Shanahan 2003, 69)

- poor glycemic control
- loss of sensation of the feet
- decreased perspiration
- lack of attention to the feet and nails
- previous history of ulceration
- structural deformity
- limited joint range of motion
- obesity
- diabetes of 15 years or longer
- smoking
- alcohol use

Clinical Signs

- callus build-up on the plantar surface of the foot (also referred to as a "hot spot") (Figures 10–3 and 10–4; Color Plates 21 and 22)
- ulceration over the metatarsal heads or the plantar surface of the hallux (heel)
- ulceration on the plantar surface of foot deformity (often with a punched out appearance)
- cracks in the skin between the toes or at the base of the toes on the plantar surface of the foot

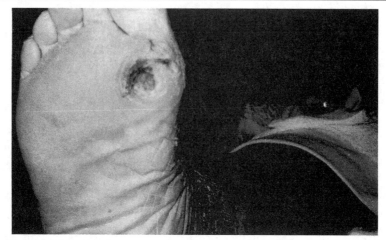

Figure 10–3 Diabetic Ulcer Needs Saucer-Style Debridement of Callus. Note dry skin at ankle, typical of diabetics.

Clinical Objectives:
(1) Clean
(2) Keep moist
(3) Manage exudate
(4) Eliminate pressure (non–weight bearing)
See Color Plate 21.

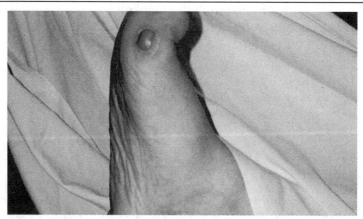

Figure 10–4 Diabetic Foot Ulcer with Hypergranulation Tissue, Callus Margin.

Clinical Objectives:
(1) Clean
(2) Keep moist
(3) Manage exudate
(4) Eliminate pressure
See Color Plate 22.

Ulcer

Assess the ulcer for

- location
- length, width, and depth
  - The NPUAP staging system for pressure ulcers can be used (Exhibit 6–1, page 96).
  - Wagner scale for diabetic foot ulcers (Exhibit 10–1, this page).
  - partial thickness and full thickness (see Chapter 2, Assessment and Documentation for Wounds)
- exudate (color and amount)
- erythema (around the ulcer)
- edema (in the tissue around the ulcer)
- wound bed (percent of the wound bed with granulation, yellow devitalized tissue, and black eschar)
- odor
- suspected or confirmed infection
- undermining
- length of time the patient has had the ulcer

Check the foot for loss of protective sensation (Exhibit 10–2, page 186).

- presence or absence of pulses (dorsalis pedis, posterior tibialis)
- location of deformities
- condition of the toes and nails (who trims the nails and how)
- condition of the skin, including the presence and locations of calluses, cracks, and fissures
- sensory examination using a Semmes-Weinstein monfilament
  - The patient should be supine or sitting with feet supported. (Exhibit 10–2.)

Exhibit 10–1 Wagner Scale

Grade	Description
Grade 0	Skin intact
Grade 1	Superficial ulcer
Grade 2	Deeper ulcer to tendon or bone
Grade 3	Ulcer has abscess or osteomyelitis
Grade 4	Gangrene on forefoot
Grade 5	Gangrene over major portion of foot

Exhibit 10–2 Management of the Insensitive Foot in Diabetes

DIABETIC FOOT SCREEN	Date: _____
Patient's Name (Last, First, Middle) _____	ID No.:_____

Fill in the following blanks with an "R," "L," or "B" to indicate positive findings on the right, left, or both feet.

Has there been a change in the foot since last evaluation?   Yes ___   No ___

Is there a foot ulcer now or history of foot ulcer?   Yes ___   No ___

Does the foot have an abnormal shape?   Yes ___   No ___

Is there weakness in the ankle or foot?   Yes ___   No ___

Are the nails thick, too long, or ingrown?   Yes ___   No ___

Label sensory level with a "+" in the circled areas of the foot if the patient can feel the 10-gram (5.07 Semmes-Weinstein) nylon filament and "–" if he/she cannot feel the 10-gram filament.

Callus▨   Pre-ulcer▧   Ulcer■ (note with/depth in cm)

and label skin condition with R—Redness, S—Swelling, W—Warmth, D—Dryness, M—Maceration

Vascular:	Brachial Systolic Pressure	R_____	L_____
	Ankle Systolic Pressure	R_____	L_____
	Ischemic Index	R_____	L_____

Does the patient use footwear appropriate for his/her category?   Yes___   No___

RISK CATEGORY:

_____   0   No loss of protective sensation.

_____   1   Loss of protective sensation with no weakness, deformity, callus, pre-ulcer or history of ulceration.

_____   2   Loss of protective sensation with weakness, deformity, pre-ulcer or callus but no history of ulceration; or Ischemic Index < 0.45.

_____   3   History of plantar ulceration.

- The patient should be able to identify the area on the plantar surface of the foot being touched with the monofilament.
- type of footwear used and how long the patient has been wearing the current shoes
- who inspects the feet for the patient and how often
- history of previous foot ulcerations/amputations

Complications

- deepening of the ulcer to the tendons and bone
- infection
    - Signs include increased amounts of drainage, erythema, pain, temperature, foul odor, and red streaks running up the leg from the ulcer.
    - This is a common complication that progresses to gangrene.
    - Best management depends on a early diagnosis, appropriate antibiotic therapy, and surgical debridement.
- gangrene
- amputation

TREATMENT CHOICES

Management of the Ulcer

- radiographic imaging to rule out osteomyelitis, foreign objects, and asymptomatic fractures
- debridement to remove necrotic tissue and determine the ulcer depth
- revascularization for those with limb threatening arterial insufficiency
- biopsy for ulcers in an uncommon location
- aggressive antibiotic coverage when infection is present (Most common pathogens are aerobic, gram-positive staphylococci and streptococci, although other pathogens can be present, including anaerobes.)
- avoidance of weight bearing (Walking on the ulcer can cause further necrosis, delay healing, and force bacteria into deeper tissues. The best method is considered to be the total-contact cast—contraindicated for foot ulcers with abscess, osteomyelitis, or a similar deep infection or gangrene.) (Figure 10–5)
- adequate nutrition including vitamins, minerals, protein, and good glucose control

- topical dressing chosen according to the location, size, depth, amount of drainage, and type of wound (The selection of a topical dressing without including the other items listed above increases the probability of an amputation.)

TIPS • Even though it may look as though there is not an ulcer under a callus, it needs to be evaluated by an expert in your community (e.g., podiatrist, diabetic foot specialist).
- An ulcer that appears shallow can extend deep into the tissues of the foot.
- This is not the type of ulcer on which to try first one type of dressing and then another, thinking you will find a magical fix by the appropriate choice of a topical treatment. This ulcer needs aggressive treatment by someone who routinely treats diabetic foot ulcers.
- Lawsuits commonly result from amputations; providing appropriate care and referral is essential.

PREVENTION

Management of Healed Ulcers

- Prevention of friction and callus build-up requires proper orthodics/therapeutic footwear.

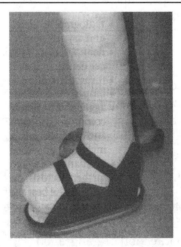

Figure 10–5 Total-Contact Cast.

- Those with Charcot foot need a molded shoe.
- Podiatrists and/or certified pedorthists are qualified for the proper fitting of therapeutic shoes and insoles. See Exhibit 10–3 for Medicare guidelines.
- Those with peripheral neuropathy, peripheral arterial disease, previous ulceration, or deformed feet are discouraged from jogging, prolonged walking, and treadmill exercises.
- Daily foot inspection by the patient or caregiver is vital.

Patient Education

- importance of foot care (Exhibits 10–4, page 192, and 10–5, page 193)
- control of blood sugar

NAIL CARE (Kelechi and Lukas 1997)

- The goal depends upon the patient, but generally includes improving comfort, reducing embarrassment from unattractive nails, and making the shoes less painful.
- Instructions on proper assessment and trimming are needed as trimming dystrophic nails is considered debridement.
- Controversy exists in the literature on the best method of debriding nails. The overall result should be a smooth nail border without sharp edges in the corners.
- The nurse must always remember to wear gloves and a mask, and in some cases a gown, for protection from contaminants that are harbored under the nails and become airborne.
- Interventions include the following (Kelechi and Lukas, *Basic Foot Care: A Self-Instruction Manual*, 1999, p. 53):
  - Assess overall hygiene, circulation, sensation, skin, toenails, mobility, condition of the footwear, and level of patient understanding.
  - Trimming nails includes the appropriate tools—a spring barrel nail nipper and emery board or pumice stone.
  - Basic foot care includes washing and drying the feet and applying an emollient; however, emollients should not be placed between the toes.
  - Corns, calluses, and dystrophic nails should be cared for by a nurse who has been taught nail debridement or by a physician or podiatrist.

Exhibit 10–3 Medicare Coverage of Therapeutic Footwear for People with Diabetes

Medicare provides coverage for depth-inlay shoes, custom-molded shoes, and shoe inserts for people with diabetes who qualify under Medicare Part B. Designed to prevent lower-limb ulcers and amputations in people who have diabetes, this Medicare benefit can prevent suffering and save money.

HOW INDIVIDUALS QUALIFY

The MD or DO treating the patient for diabetes must certify that the individual:

1. has diabetes

2. has one or more of the following conditions in one or both feet:

   - history of partial or complete foot amputation
   - history of previous foot ulceration
   - history of pre-ulcerative callus
   - peripheral neuropathy with evidence of callus formation
   - poor circulation
   - foot deformity

3. is being treated under a comprehensive diabetes care plan and needs therapeutic shoes and/or inserts because of diabetes

TYPE OF FOOTWEAR COVERED

If an individual qualifies, he/she is limited to one of the following footwear categories within one calendar year:

1. one pair of depth-inlay shoes and three pairs of inserts

2. one pair of custom-molded shoes (including inserts) and two additional pairs of inserts

Separate inserts may be covered under certain criteria. Shoe modification is covered as a substitute for an insert, and a custom-molded shoe is covered when the individual has a foot deformity that cannot be accommodated by a depth shoe.

WHAT THE PHYSICIAN NEEDS TO DO

1. The **certifying physician** (the MD or DO) overseeing the diabetes treatment must review and sign a Statement of Certifying Physician for Therapeutic Shoes.

continues

Exhibit 10–3 continued

2. The **prescribing physician** (the DPM, orthopaedic foot surgeon, or MD) must complete a footwear prescription. Once the patient has the **signed statement and the prescription,** he/she can see a podiatrist, orthotist, prosthetist, or pedorthist to have the prescription filled. The supplier will then submit the Medicare claim form (Form HCFA 1500) to the appropriate durable medical equipment regional carrier (DMERC), keeping copies of the claim form and the original statement and prescription.

Note that in most cases the certifying physician and the prescribing physician will be two different individuals.

PATIENT RESPONSIBILITY FOR PAYMENT

Medicare will pay for 80 percent of the payment amount allowed either directly to the patient or by reimbursement. The patient is responsible for a minimum of 20 percent of the total payment amount and possibly more if the dispenser does not accept Medicare assignment and if the dispenser's usual fee is higher than the payment amount. The maximum payment amount per pair as of 1997 is listed below. These figures may change.

	Total Amount Allowed	Amount Covered by Medicare
Depth-inlay shoes	$126.00	$100.80
Custom-molded shoes	378.00	302.40
Inserts or modifications	64.00	51.20

THE PEDORTHIC DISPENSER

Properly fitting therapeutic footwear requires special skills and care. The pedorthic profession focuses on the design, fit, and modification of shoes and related foot appliances. For a listing of pedorthists, send a self-addressed stamped envelope to the Board for Certification in Pedorthics, 9861 Broken Land Pkwy, #255, Columbia, MD 21046.

Exhibit 10–4 Patient Guide: Care of the Diabetic Foot

- Do not smoke.
- Inspect the feet daily for blisters, cuts, and scratches. The use of a mirror can aid in seeing the bottom of the feet. Always check between the toes.

continues

Exhibit 10–4 continued

- Wash feet daily. Dry carefully, especially between the toes.

- Avoid extremes of temperatures. Test water with hand, elbow, or thermometer before bathing.

- If feet feel cold at night, wear socks. Do not apply hot water bottles or heating pads. Do not use an electric blanket. Do not soak feet in hot water.

- Do not walk on hot surfaces, such as sandy beaches or on cement around swimming pools.

- Do not walk barefoot.

- Do not use chemical agents for removal of corns and calluses, corn plasters, or strong antiseptic solutions.

- Do not use adhesive tape on the feet.

- Inspect the inside of shoes daily for foreign objects, nail points, torn linings, and rough areas.

- If vision is impaired, have a family member inspect feet daily, trim nails, and buff calluses.

- For dry feet, use a very thin coat of a lubricating oil or cream. Apply this after bathing and drying feet. Do not put the oil or cream between the toes. Consult your physician for detailed instructions.

- Stockings: Wear properly fitting stockings. Do not wear mended stockings or stockings with seams. Change stockings daily.

- Do not wear garters.

- Shoes should be comfortable at the time of purchase. Do not depend on them to stretch out. Shoes should be made of leather. Purchase shoes late in the afternoon when feet are the largest. Running or special walking shoes may be worn after checking with your physician. Purchase shoes from shoe sales people who understand diabetic foot problems.

- Do not wear shoes without stockings.

- Do not wear sandals with thongs between the toes.

- In winter time, take special precautions. Wear wool socks and protective foot gear such as fleece-lined boots.

- Cut nails straight across.

- Do not cut corns and calluses: follow instructions from your physician or podiatrist.

- Avoid crossing your legs: this can cause pressure on the nerves.

- See your physician regularly and be sure that your feet are examined at each visit.

- Notify your physician or podiatrist at once should you develop a blister or sore on your feet.

- Be sure to inform your podiatrist that you are a diabetic.

Exhibit 10–5 Teaching Guide: Charcot Joints

WHAT ARE CHARCOT JOINTS?

In the late 1800s, a French physician, Dr. J.M. Charcot, first described the destructive changes in the joints of people with decreased feeling in their legs and feet. Today, the term Charcot joint is used to refer to any joint in the insensate foot that is destroyed or dislocated. The term Charcot foot is used to refer to a foot with many Charcot joints that has actually changed shape.

There is usually not a single event or major injury to the insensate foot that causes fractures or destruction of the joints, but an accumulation of many small injuries that result in Charcot joints or a Charcot foot.

FACTORS THAT WILL INCREASE THE CHANCE OF DEVELOPING A CHARCOT JOINT

- loss of protective sensation
- activities or conditions that put increased stress on the feet
- shoes that do not provide support

WHAT CAUSES CHARCOT JOINTS?

Feet, with or without feeling, experience injury or trauma every day as a normal part of walking. The difference between the insensate foot and one with feeling is that injury will cause the person with feeling to stop walking to rest or protect the injured foot. The person with insensate feet will continue to walk, causing further injury with possible bone and joint destruction.

Muscle strength in the feet and legs of a person without sensation is usually decreased as part of the disease process. This loss leads to a muscle imbalance affecting how a person walks and the way the foot functions. The foot will strike the ground harder during walking, resulting in greater impact to the bones and joints, causing greater and more frequent injury. Twists or sprains of the foot and ankle are more common, and even though there is significant injury, the person without sensation will continue to use the foot.

Another complication occurring with the insensate foot is a loss of muscle tone in the blood vessels supplying blood to the feet. This results in increased blood flow, which can remove some of the minerals that normally keep bones strong. Weakened bones are more likely to break when stressed.

WHAT DOES THIS MEAN TO A PERSON WITH AN INSENSATE FOOT?

In the insensate foot, pain that would warn a person with normal sensation of injury is not present. You need to be aware of other signs that an injury has occurred. If a bone is broken or a Charcot joint has occurred, you will have one or all of the following signs:

- swelling (mild or great)

continues

Exhibit 10–5 continued

- an increase in skin temperature in the area
- redness in the area
- a lack of sweating, resulting in dryness of the skin over the area

Some patients wait until a fifth sign appears: destruction and structural change (the foot appears shorter and wider). An untreated Charcot foot develops a "rocker bottom" shape much like a rocker on a rocking chair. The arch of the foot collapses and joints are destroyed.

TREATMENT

The best treatment is prevention:

- Insensate feet need special attention; visit your physician regularly.
- Insensate feet need support, protection, and cushioning to help prevent fractures and movement of the bones. This includes special footwear, extra-depth shoes, molded insoles, and special custom-made shoes.
- Inspect your feet daily.

If prevention fails and the signs of Charcot joints appear, seek medical attention IMMEDIATELY to determine the severity. If a fracture has occurred, healing will include protecting the foot from further injury. Forms of protection may involve any of the following:

- casts
- wheelchair
- crutches
- bed rest

Sometimes joint destruction is severe enough to result in a permanently misshapen foot with bony bumps or prominences. This condition will always require special shoes. Sometimes surgery to fuse broken joints or remove bony prominences may be necessary.

CASE STUDY

Joseph Alexander, who is 66 years old, obese, and a smoker, was referred to your agency from the Centerville Hospital following a brief hospitalization for poor blood glucose control and a foot infection. He had stepped on an unknown object and developed an ulcer on his left foot. While in the hospital, he received diabetic dietary instruction, and he was placed on intravenous antibiotic therapy for the infection that had resulted from the injury. He was discharged on oral antibiotics. Joseph, an insulin-dependent diabetic for 20 years, had developed peripheral neuropathy and was unaware when or how he injured his foot. He noticed blood on his sock, put a bandage on the spot, and had forgotten about it. When he had his feet up one evening watching television, his wife noticed the redness that was developing on the bottom (plantar surface) of his foot. She insisted he see the physician, which had resulted in his hospitalization. During the admission interview, you discover Joseph has no understanding of regular foot checks or of diabetic foot care. He purchases his shoes at the local discount store, but tells you they have never been uncomfortable (remember he has peripheral neuropathy). When you examine Joseph's feet, you discover a callus on the first metatarsal head (bottom of the foot below the great toe, commonly referred to as the ball of the foot) on the right foot. There is no discoloration, erythema, or exudate from the area. His toes on both feet are beginning to have a cocked up appearance. His toenails on both feet are jagged, thick, and yellowed. Joseph tells you his feet are becoming flat although you do not see any erythema or swelling at the arch of either of his feet. They are not hot to the touch, which is a symptom of stage 1 in the development of acute Charcot inflammation. You are able to palpate pulses in both feet. The ulcer on the left foot is located on the heel (hallux) of his foot. The wound base is 80 percent yellow, devitalized tissue and 20 percent granulation. There is 1.0 cm of erythema surrounding the 2.0 cm long × 1.5 cm wide ulcer. You are unable to tell the true depth of the ulcer due to the presence of the devitalized tissue; however, it is currently 0.5 cm deep. There is no odor, and the alginate dressing applied the day before is saturated with sanguineous exudate.

When you are presented with this or a similar case, there are a multitude of issues to address. Remember when you are putting these issues in priority, not all physicians are diabetic specialists or understand the complexities of the diabetic foot. Who, in your area, are your referral sources for care of the diabetic foot ulcer, nail care, and footwear? The patient described above has had a course of intravenous antibiotics, but not aggressive treatment of the ulcer. One short course of antibiotics is not the only treatment for this patient nor is a topical dressing that provides autolytic debridement. Infection is a common and quick complication, and the ulcer needs aggressive debridement, X-rays to see if there is osteomyelitis present, and off-loading of the pressure. During the course of treatment for the ulcer, he will also need education on the care of his feet and nails, assessment of his understanding of nutrition and glucose control, callus removal from the right foot, and appropriate footwear.

After the ulcer is healed on the left foot, he will need appropriate footwear for the left foot as well. As mentioned at the beginning of this chapter, care of the diabetic patient is complex. This is an overview of some of the main concerns of the patient with a diabetic foot ulcer. Prepare before you meet this patient by finding out who your resources are: diabetic specialists, foot clinics, podiatrists, and/or pedorthists.

REFERENCES

Armstrong, D. G. et al. 1998. Risk factors for diabetic foot ulceration: A logical approach to treatment. *Journal of Wound, Ostomy, and Continence Nursing* 25(3), 123–128.

Elftman, P. 1998. Management of the neuropathic foot. In *Wound care: A collaborative practice manual for physical therapists and nurses.* eds. C. Sussman and B. M. Bates-Jensen, 315–345. Gaithersburg, MD: Aspen Publishers, Inc.

Kelechi, T. J., and Lukas, K. S. 1997. Options in practice: Patient with dystrophic toenails, calluses, and heel fissures. *Journal of Wound, Ostomy, and Continence Nursing* 24(4), 237–242.

Kelechi, T. J., and Lukas, K. S. 1999. *Basic foot care: A self-instructional manual.* Charleston, SC: Center for the Study of Aging, Medical University of South Carolina.

Kravitz, S. R., McGuire, J., & Shanahan, S. D. 2003. Physical assessment of the diabetic foot. *Advances in Skin & Wound Care* 16(2), 68–75.

Lavery, L. A., Baranoski, S., & Ayello, E. A. 2000. Diabetic foot ulcers. In S. Baranoski and E. A. Ayello (Eds.), *Wound care essentials: Practice principles* (311–332). Philadelphia, PA: Lippincott Williams & Wilkins.

Levin, M. E. 1998. Prevention and treatment of diabetic foot wounds. *Journal of Wound, Ostomy, and Continence Nursing* 25(3), 129–146.

Levin, M. E. et al. (Eds.) 1993. *The diabetic foot*, 5th ed. St. Louis, MO: Mosby Year Book.

Mulder, G. A. 2000. Evaluating and managing the diabetes foot: An overview. *Advances in Skin and Wound Care* 13(1), 33–39.

Steed, D. L. 1997. Diabetic wounds: Assessment, classification and management. In *Chronic wound care: A clinical source book for healthcare professionals*, eds. D. Krasner and D. Kane, 172–177. Wayne, PA: Health Management Publications.

Synder, R. S., Cohen, M. M., Sevin, C., and Livingston, J. 2001. Osteomyelitis in the diabetic patient: Diagnosis and treatment part I: Overview, diagnosis and microbiology. *Ostomy Wound Management* 47(1), 18–30.

BIBLIOGRAPHY

Frykberg, R. G. 1998. The team approach in diabetic foot management. *Advances in Wound Care* 11(2), 71–77.

Levin, M. E. 1997. Diabetic foot wounds: Pathogenesis and management. *Advances in Wound Care* 10(2), 24–30.

RESOURCES

National Diabetes Education Program: Feet Can Last a Lifetime; Internet: http://www.ndep.nih.gov/materials/pubs/feet/feet.htm

National Diabetes Information Clearinghouse (NDIC), 1 Information Way, Bethesda, MD 20892-3560; Internet: http://www.niddk.nih.gov; 1-800-GET-LEVEL

American Diabetes Association, 1660 Duke St., Alexandria, VA 22314; Internet: http://www. diabetes.org.ada

American Association of Diabetic Educators, 444 N. Michigan Avenue, Suite 1240, Chicago, IL 60611-3901; Internet: http://www.aadenet.org

Teresa Kelechi, Center for the Study of Aging, Medical University of South Carolina, 171 Ashley Avenue, Charleston, SC 29425

Wound, Ostomy and Continence Nurses Society. 2004. Guidelines for managment of wounds in patients with lower-extremity neuropathic disease. Glenview, IL. Author.

CHAPTER 11

Skin Tears

Donna Oddo

Skin tears are a common problem in wound care. Minor skin tears can be resolved with minimal intervention. Serious skin tears may lead to large areas of skin loss, fluid imbalances, infections, and sepsis. Long-term complex care, possibly even skin grafts, could be required to achieve closure. They often cause disfigurement and altered body image concerns. Although skin tears may occur anywhere on the body, they are most commonly seen on the upper extremities. It is important to correctly identify and document skin tears and not place them in the category of a pressure ulcer. (Figures 11–1 and 11–2; Color Plates 8 and 23)

Skin tears are most likely to occur on fragile, aged, dry skin. They can be caused by trauma, such as a bump or fall, or by removal of adhesives on the skin. When treating skin tears, caution must be taken to avoid further skin damage by minimizing the use of adhesives.

ETIOLOGY

In normal tissue, dermal and epidermal tissue are firmly meshed. In aging skin, there is

- decreased collagen
- decreased elasticity
- decreased epidermis thickness
- decreased turgor
- decreased subcutaneous fat

ASSESSMENT

There are four types of tears:

1. flaps
    *   viable—integrity restored
    *   nonviable—tissue loss results
2. linear (epidermal tissue that can be approximated without loss of coverage)
3. partial-thickness tissue loss (tissue loss involving the epidermis and into but not through the dermis)
4. full-thickness tissue loss (unusual; extends through the epidermis and dermis and into the subcutaneous tissue)

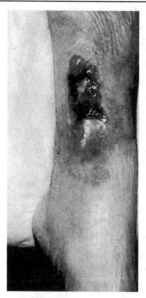

Figure 11–1 Skin Tear on Lower Extremity. Note fragile "onion peel" type skin surrounding the wound.

Clinical Objectives:

(1) Clean

(2) Protect wound and surrounding tissue

(3) Keep moist

See Color Plate 8.

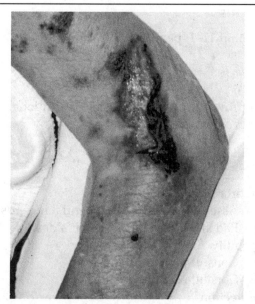

Figure 11–2 Skin Tear with 75 Percent of Epidermal Flap Missing.
Clinical Objectives:
(1) Approximate the skin tear flap/tissue as closely as possible
(2) Protect wound and surrounding tissue
(3) Keep moist
(4) No tape on skin—nonadherent dressings should be secured with a gauze or tubular nonadhesive wrap.
See Color Plate 23.

PREVENTION

Patients at Risk

- elderly
- frail
- previous skin tears
- poor nutritional status
- poor hydration status
- poor mobility
- dementia
- history of falls
- history of bruising

Interventions

See Exhibit 11–1, page 203.

Intrinsic

- Improve nutritional status (see nutritional exhibits in Chapter 4).
- Improve hydration status.

Extrinsic

- environment
  - Assess living area for potential hazards.
  - Pad side rails or wheelchair sides.
- mobility
  - Consult physical therapy.
  - Consult occupational therapy.
- protection
  - Moisturize skin.
  - Use sleeves or stockinette.

Education

(See Exhibit 11–2, page 205).

- nutrition and hydration
- safety issues
- protection

TREATMENT CHOICES

Goals

- Prevent further tears.
- Maintain an environment to promote wound healing.

Flaps (Viable) or Linear Tears

- Steri-strips—Use caution if more than 24 hours have passed from time of injury or if the injury involved contamination of tissue with "dirty" object.

Exhibit 11–1 How to Stop Skin Tears

Soften the skin; use moisturizers liberally.

Treat new tears promptly.

Optimize the host—a healthy patient is less likely to experience tears.

Protect the arms with sleeves or stockinette.

Safety-check environment for sharp edges, fall hazards.

Keep needed items in reach of patient.

Instruct patient and caregivers in home safety and skin care.

No aggressive adhesives on fragile skin!

Transfer with caution; protect fragile skin from friction.

Encourage fluids.

Assess need for multidisciplinary interventions.

Reevaluate frequently.

Skin tears are preventable!

- Transparent film—Use only if drainage is minimal and the wound is clean.

Partial Thickness Skin Tears

- Antibiotic ointment and nonadherent dressing
- Foam dressing—useful when decreasing frequency of dressing changes, minimizes trauma to surrounding tissue

Full Thickness Skin Tears

- Hydrogel impregnated gauze
- Alginates
- Foams
- Surgical intervention (grafting)

CASE STUDY

Mrs. Peters is an 86-year-old white female referred to home health for assessment and management of skin tears on her bilateral upper extremities. They were sustained after a fall in her bathroom.

Examination revealed a frail, thin woman with poor turgor and very dry skin. She was unkempt, stating "my daughter has been taking care of me, but she died last month. I'm not doing too well on my own." Mrs. Peters has a history of mild congestive heart failure for which she took digoxin and furosemide daily.

Dressings (gauze wrap) covered both arms and were held fast to her skin with dried sanguineous drainage. To ease removal and lessen trauma to the skin, the dressings were soaked in saline. On the right forearm, a linear tear was noted, measuring 3 cm long × 4 cm wide × 0 deep. The surrounding skin was intact, but with a fragile "onion skin" appearance. The left forearm revealed a partial thickness tear 4 cm long × 3 cm wide × 2 cm deep. Neither wound was actively bleeding, nor was there any erythema, warmth, or induration. Both sites were cleansed with normal saline, and the intact skin was treated with a protective skin barrier wipe. A transparent film dressing was placed over the linear tear on the right arm. A nonadherent foam dressing was placed over the wound on the left arm and secured in place with gauze wrap. Tubed gauze was applied to both arms for protection from wrist to above the elbow. A plan of care was established for Mrs. Peters using an interdisciplinary approach. The nurse continued to visit, changing the transparent film dressing weekly, and changing the foam dressing three times weekly. The nurse also drew blood for analysis.

Mrs. Peters was then instructed, per physician order, to lower her dose of digoxin and add a potassium supplement. She was taught signs and symptoms of electrolyte imbalance and digoxin toxicity. Her diet teaching stressed the importance of adequate protein, calories, and potassium-rich foods. A home health aide visited three times weekly to assist with personal care and to moisturize Mrs. Peters's dry skin. A physical therapist developed an exercise regimen to help strengthen the patient and enhance her mobility. A walker and a raised toilet seat were obtained; the towel bar (where the left arm injury occurred) was removed as were skid rugs in the bathroom. A social worker assisted with community resources and arranging for private assistance after discharge from home health.

Mrs. Peters was discharged from home health following 6 weeks of care. Both skin tears had healed, no new tears occurred. She was more mobile, safer, and more secure in her own abilities. A support system had been established within the community.

Exhibit 11–2 Patient Guide: Preventing and Treating Skin Tears

---

Aging, certain illnesses, and medications may cause the skin to become dry and fragile. When this happens, any bump or minor injury may cause the skin to open or tear. These skin tears may bleed, become infected, or lead to more serious skin problems. If this is a new problem, seek medical advice to determine the cause of the skin changes.

The following measures may reduce the risk of getting skin tears:

- Eat a well-balanced diet.
- Drink plenty of fluids, especially water.
- Keep skin soft and supple by using only mild soap and by applying a moisturizing cream daily.
- If experiencing balance problems or falls, seek medical advice regarding the cause and about the use of medical equipment to keep you safe (such as walkers or canes).
- Check the home for any sharp hazards. Keep pathways clear.
- Use extra caution in the bathroom. Consider installing grab bars where needed.
- Consider wearing long sleeves to protect your arms.

If you do experience a skin tear, the following measures may be taken:

- Cleanse the wound with mild soap and water. Rinse well with plain water. Pat dry gently with gauze or a clean washcloth.
- Stop the bleeding by applying gentle pressure with gauze or a clean washcloth.
- Apply an antibiotic ointment sparingly to the open wound bed.
- Cover with a nonstick gauze pad.
- Change the dressing each day, cleaning each time with mild soap and water.
- If the wound involves a large area of skin, if the bleeding does not stop quickly, or if signs of infection develop, seek medical advice. Signs of infection include redness and warmth surrounding the wound, change in the color of the drainage, foul odor, fever, or increased discomfort at the site.

BIBLIOGRAPHY

Baranoski, S. 2000. Skin tears: The enemy of frail skin. *Advances in Skin & Wound Care* 13(3), 123–126.

Krasner, D., and D. Kane, eds. 1997. *Chronic wound care: A clinical source book for healthcare professionals*, 2d ed. Wayne, PA: Health Management Publications.

McGough-Csarny, J. 1998. Skin tears in institutionalized elderly: An epidemiological study. *Ostomy/Wound Management* 44(3A), 145–255.

Pieper, B. et al. 1999. Wound prevalence, types and treatments in home care. *Advanced Wound Care* 12(3), 117–125.

Valdes, A. et al. 1999. A multidisciplinary, therapy-based, team approach for efficient and effective wound healing: A retrospective study. *Ostomy/Wound Management* 45(6), 30–36.

CHAPTER 12

Surgical Wounds and Radiation Burns

Pamela Brown

SURGICAL WOUNDS

Surgical wounds and lacerations are usually closed by primary intention. The wound margins (edges) are brought together soon after the wounding and secured with sutures, staples, or adhesive strips. Wounds closed by primary intention usually heal in 7–14 days with minimal scarring (Figure 12–1; Color Plate 24). Occasionally, such a wound fails to heal properly, resulting in separation of the wound margins and dehiscence or evisceration (Figures 12–2 and 12–3; Color Plates 25 and 26). These wounds are usually left open to heal by secondary intention. The wound edges contract and decrease the size of the wound while the wound bed fills in with granulation (scar) tissue. Finally epithelization of the wound surface occurs. This process may take weeks or months. (See Table 12–1, page 210, and Exhibits 12–1, page 212, and 12–2, page 213).

Cleaning the Wound

The surgical wound must be cleansed with each dressing change. Use normal saline with an angiocath and syringe to thoroughly irrigate the wound. A spray saline that can provide a therapeutic pressure or a nonionic surfactant wound cleanser can also be used.

Treatment Choices

Frequency of dressing change depends on the amount and type of wound drainage. The manufacturer's recommendations for products used should be followed.

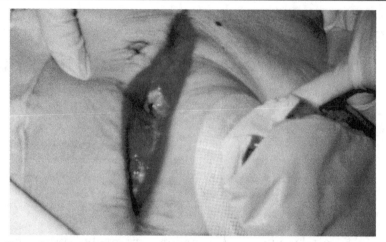

Figure 12–1 Clean, Granular Surgical Wound with Small Amount of Slough in Center. Note colostomy.

   Clinical Objectives:

   (1) Clean

   (2) Keep moist

   (3) Manage exudate

   (4) Protect from colostomy drainage

   See Color Plate 24.

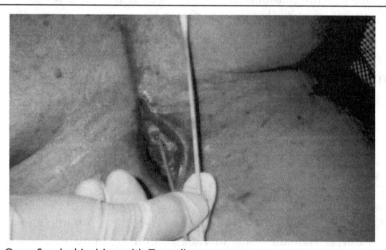

Figure 12–2 Open Surgical Incision with Tunneling.

   Clinical Objectives:

   (1) Clean

   (2) Keep moist

   (3) Manage exudate

   (4) Pack tunneling loosely

   See Color Plate 25.

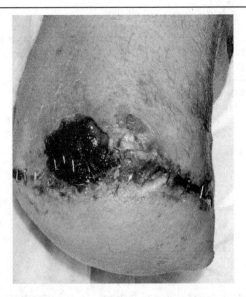

Figure 12–3 Necrotic Tissue (Eschar) at Above-Knee Amputation Site of Stump Incision Line. Note erythema and poorly approximated incision line.

Clinical Objectives:

(1) Remove eschar

(2) Clean

(3) Keep moist

(4) Manage exudate

(5) Culture (if appropriate)

See Color Plate 26.

Exudating Wounds

(These wounds may or may not need debridement.)

- calcium alginate
- hydrofibers
- gauze moistened with normal saline

Nonexudating Wounds

Use a dressing that will keep the wound bed moist and clean of necrotic tissue.

- gauze moistened with normal saline
- wound gel or gauze impregnated with gel

Table 12–1 Healing Signs for Surgical Wound Healing

Outcome Measure	Days 1–4: New Wound	Days 5–9: Healing	Days 10–14: Proliferative Healing	Day 15—Years 1–2: New Skin Forming
Incision color	Red, edges approximated	Red, progressing to bright pink (all skin tones)	Bright pink (all skin tones)	Pale pink, progressing to white or silver in light-skinned patients; pale pink, progressing to darker than normal skin color or may blanch to white in dark-skinned patients.
Surrounding tissue inflammation	Swelling, redness, or skin discoloration; warmth, pain	None present	None present	None present
Drainage type	Bloody, progressing to yellow/clear	None present	None present	None present
Drainage amount	Moderate to minimal	None present	None present	None present
Closure materials	Present, may be sutures or staples	Beginning to remove external sutures/staples	Sutures/staples removed, Steri-strips or tape strips may be present	None present
New skin	Present by day 4 along entire incision	Present along entire incision	Present	Present
Healing ridge	None present	Present by day 9 along entire incision	Present along entire incision	Present

COLOR PLATES

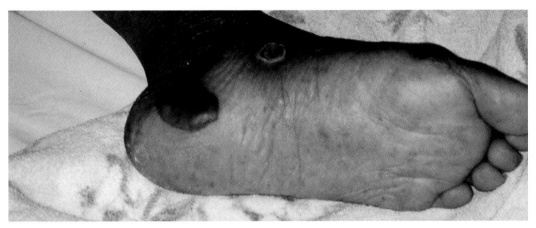

Color Plate 1 Intact Purple Heel Blister.

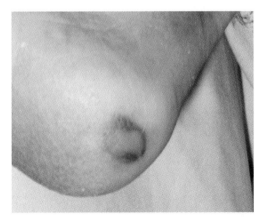

Color Plate 2 Intact Heel Blister Resolving.

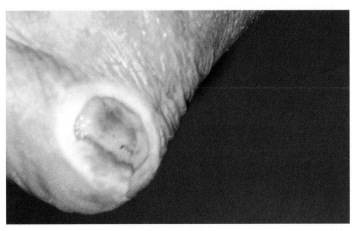

Color Plate 3 Heel Ulcer with Yellow Slough. Periwound skin macerated due to inappropriate topical treatment.

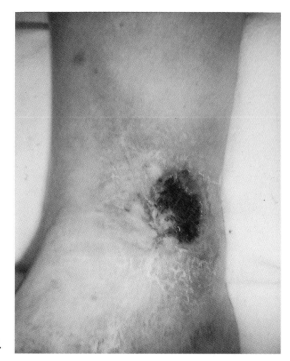

Color Plate 4 Eschar on Wound Bed.

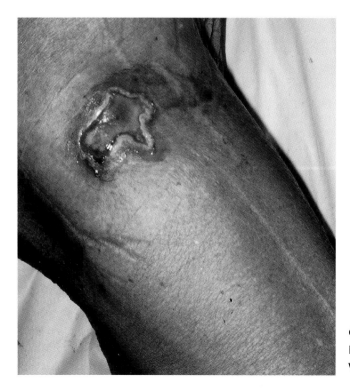

Color Plate 5 Autolytic Debridement in Progress: Slough Wound Base.

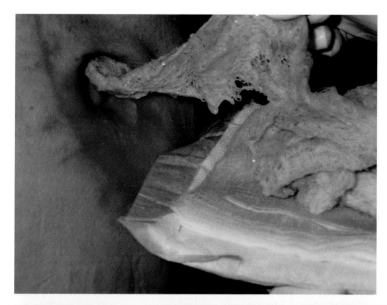

Color Plate 6 Chest Tube Site with Copious Purulent Drainage on Gauze Packing.

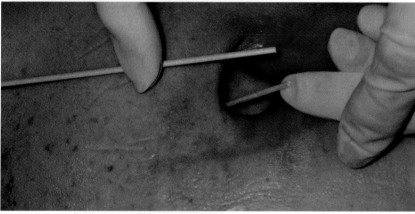

Color Plate 7 Chest Tube Site (Same as Previous Picture) with Large Tunnel.

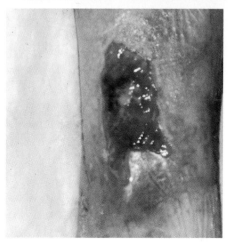

Color Plate 8 Skin Tear with Hypergranulation Tissue. Note fragile "onion peel" type skin surrounding the wound.

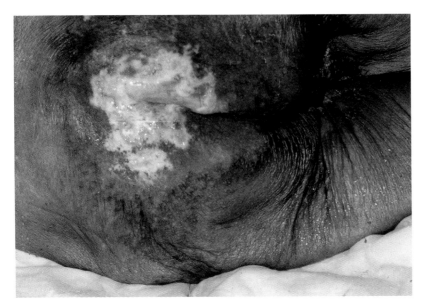

Color Plate 9
Pressure Ulcer on
Sacrum. Necrotic
center consistent
with deeper tissue
damage.

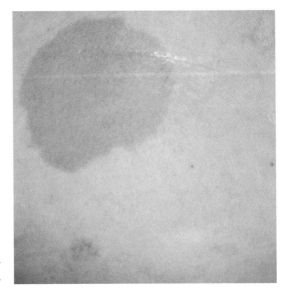

Color Plate 10 Stage I Pressure Ulcer.
Nonblanchable erythema.

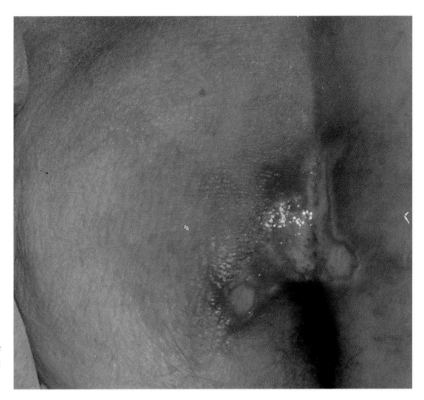

Color Plate 11
Stage II Pressure
Ulcer at Sacral
Region.

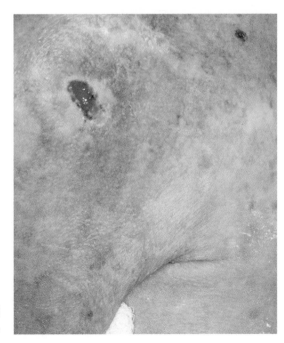

Color Plate 12 Healing
Stage III Pressure Ulcer.

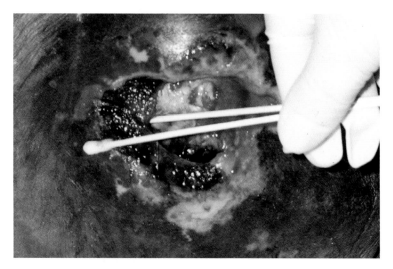

Color Plate 13 Stage IV Pressure Ulcer on Sacrum with Necrotic Tissue and Undermining.

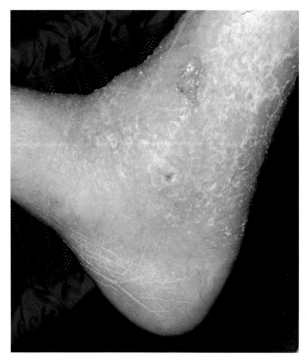

Color Plate 14 Arterial Ulcers. Note dry, flaky skin and absence of hair.

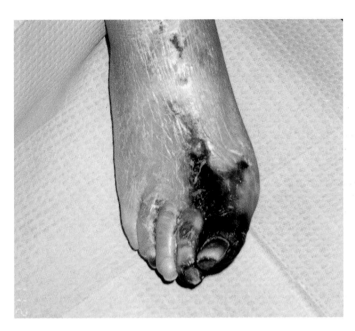

Color Plate 15 Ischemic Foot with Gangrene. Do not initiate topical treatment. Notify physician of status and any changes immediately.

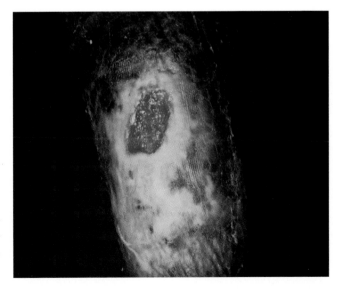

Color Plate 16 Full-Thickness Venous Stasis Ulcer on Dark-Skinned Person. Healed skin will remain light.

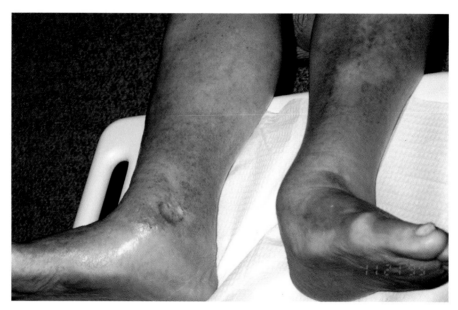

Color Plate 17 Venus Stasis Ulcer, Right Medial Ankle. Note edema, gaiter staining, and closed wound on left leg.

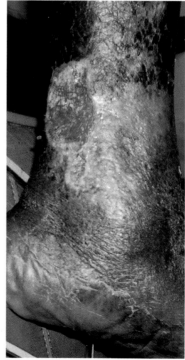

Color Plate 18 Venous Stasis Ulcer. Shallow wound bed, irregular shape, wound bed ruddy red with some yellow slough.

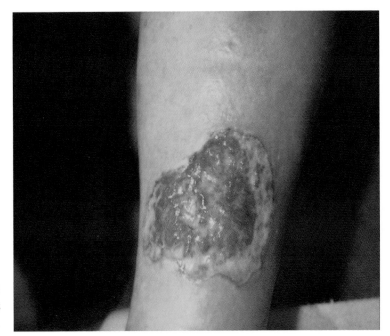

Color Plate 19 Ulcer with Mixed Disease. Patient is not a surgical candidate.

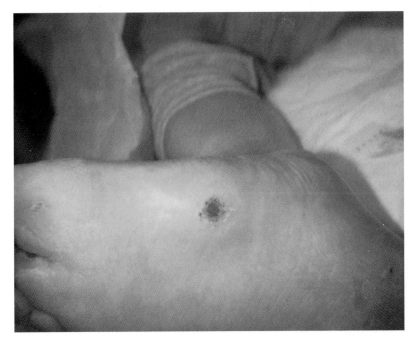

Color Plate 20 Neuropathic Ulcer; Charcot Foot.

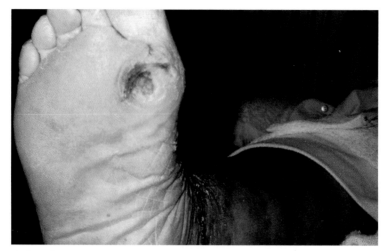

Color Plate 21 Diabetic Ulcer Needs Saucer-Style Debridement of Callus. Note dry skin at ankle, typical of diabetics.

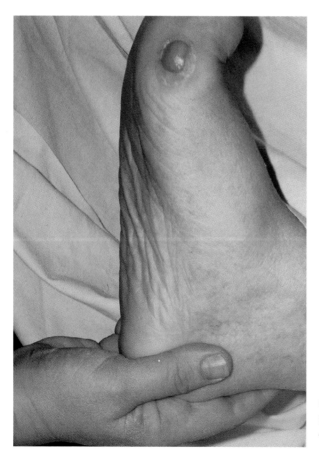

Color Plate 22 Diabetic Foot Ulcer with Hypergranulation Tissue, Callus Margin.

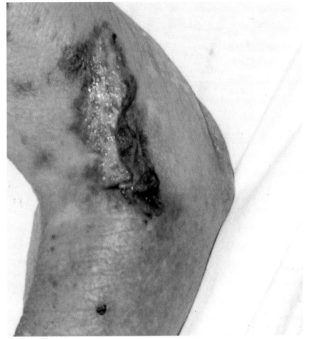

Color Plate 23 Skin Tear with 75 Percent of Epidermal Flap Missing.

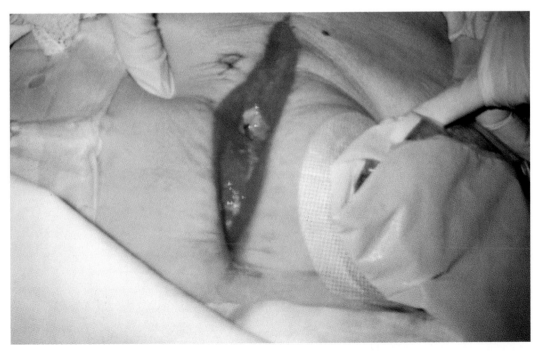

Color Plate 24 Clean, Granular Surgical Wound with Small Amount of Slough in Center. Note colostomy.

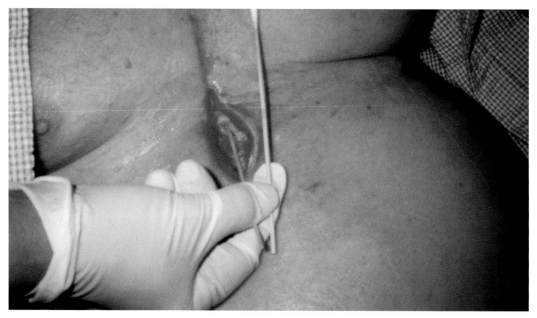

Color Plate 25 Open Surgical Incision with Tunneling.

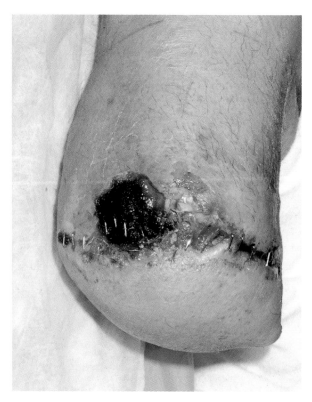

Color Plate 26 Necrotic Tissue (Eschar) at Above-Knee Amputation Site of Stump Incision Line. Note erythema and poorly approximated incision line.

Table 12–1 continued

Outcome Measure	Days 1–4: New Wound	Days 5–9: Healing	Days 10–14: Proliferative Healing	Day 15—Years 1–2: New Skin Forming
Incision	Red, edges approximated but tension evident on incision line	Red, edges may not be well approximated; tension on incision line evident	May remain red, progressing to bright pink	Prolonged new skin formation, keloid or hypertrophic scar formation
Surrounding tissue inflammation	No signs of inflammation present: no swelling, no redness or skin discoloration, no warmth, and minimal pain at incision site; hematoma (bruise) formation	Swelling, redness, or skin discoloration; warmth, pain at incision site; hematoma (bruise) formation	Prolonged inflammatory response with swelling, redness, or skin discoloration; warmth and pain; hematoma (bruising) formation	If healing, may be stalled at a plateau with no evidence of healing and continued signs of redness, pus, heat or coolness, pain or numbness
Drainage type	Bloody, progressing to yellow/clear	Red tinged/yellow and pus	Any type of drainage (pus) present	Any type of drainage (pus) present
Drainage amount	Moderate to minimal	Moderate to minimal	Any amount present	Any amount present
Closure materials	Present, may be sutures or staples	No removal of any external sutures/staples	Sutures/staples still present	For secondary intention healing, failure of wound contraction or edges not approximated
New skin	Not present along entire incision	Not present along entire incision	Not present along entire incision, opening of incision line	Not present or abnormal skin appearance, such as keloid or hypertrophic scarring
Healing ridge	None present	Not present along entire incision	Not present along entire incision, opening of incision line	Abscess formation with wound left open to heal slowly

Exhibit 12–1 Self-Care Guidelines for Acute Surgical Wound Healing

Instructions Given (Date/Initials)	Demonstration or Review of Material (Date/Initials)	Return Demonstration or States Understanding (Date/ Initials)
1. Type of incisional wound and specific cautions required		
a. No heavy lifting and other measures, to prevent hernia formation		
b. Showering or bathing area		
c. Importance of adequate nutrition for wound healing		
2. Significance of wound drainage, incision wound tissue color, surrounding tissue condition, and presence of healing ridge		
3. Wound dressing care routine:		
a. Wash hands, then remove old dressing and discard.		
b. Clean wound with normal saline.		
c. Apply primary dressing to wound.		
d. Apply secondary dressing if appropriate.		
e. Secure dressing with tape.		
f. Practice universal precautions and proper dressing disposal.		
g. Follow prescribed frequency of dressing changes.		
4. Expected change in wound appearance during healing process		
a. Scheduled removal of closure materials		
b. Incision color change as wound heals (bright red or pink to pale pink and finally to silvery white or gray)		
5. When to notify the health care provider		
a. Signs and symptoms of wound infection (erythema, edema, pain, elevated temperature, change in drainage character or amount, discoloration in tissues surrounding incision wound)		
b. Absent or incomplete healing ridge along incision after postoperative day 9 at opening of wound incision		
6. Importance of follow-up with health care provider		

Note: Must be individualized for each patient and caregiver.

TIP Older individuals are at higher risk for poorer healing outcomes. Due to physiologic changes with age, there is decreased elastin in the skin and differences in collagen replacement. The decreased rate of replacement cells affects the rate of wound healing and reepithelialization of the skin.

RADIATION BURNS

Radiation triggers changes in the skin that can create ulceration during therapy, immediately after therapy, or years after completion of radiation therapy. Radiation burns initially are shallow, and may occur spontaneously or in response to trauma. The ulcer is often painful and progressively enlarges to the margins of the irradiated skin field despite optimum treatment.

Treatment

Goals of treatment can be pain control, management of exudate, and odor control (Exhibit 12–2).

- Cleanse the wound gently with normal saline.
- Do wound care with wound gel in the form of a sheet (change daily) or amorphous hydrogel (apply three times a day) covered with a nonadherent dressing.
- Do not use tape on the skin. Use soft net, soft stretch net briefs, or tailor cotton jersey underpants or undershirts to hold the dressing in place. Do not use dressings that adhere to the wound or to the surrounding radiation-damaged skin.

Exhibit 12–2 Patient Guide: What Happens to the Skin During Radiation Therapy Treatment?

While you are receiving radiation therapy, one of the areas you and your radiation oncology team will be monitoring is your skin and the effects the radiation is having on it.

- The specific area of the body to be treated is called the treatment field.

continues

Exhibit 12–2 continued

- The cancer cells within the field are treated with radiation therapy that is administered through the skin. The skin needs special care during the treatment period.
- Radiation therapy makes the skin in the treatment field very dry. Therefore, it becomes very susceptible to skin irritations.
- The severity of skin reactions varies from person to person. One or more of the following changes can occur in the treatment field:
  - slowly increasing redness
  - dry, peeling skin
  - itching
  - swelling
  - hot sensation
  - rashes
  - blistering
  - moist, weepy areas
  - decreased perspiration
  - hair loss
  - thinning of skin

YOUR SKIN CARE IN THE TREATMENT FIELD DURING AND AFTER RADIATION THERAPY

Important: Do not remove markings on skin until instructed to do so.

Cleansing

1. Cleanse hair and body per normal routine or as recommended using mild, gentle products.
2. Use a soft washcloth to gently cleanse the treatment field—DO NOT RUB THE SKIN.
3. Rinse area and PAT dry
   Recommended shampoo, cleanser/soap: _____

Moisturizing

1. Gently apply lotion or cream to treatment field.
2. Repeat moisturizing two to three times daily.

continues

Exhibit 12–2 continued

- Use only prescribed creams or lotions in treatment field.
- Begin moisturizing after first treatment and continue as recommended. Recommended moisturizers: _____

Long-Term Care of Skin in Treatment Field

- Moisturize area every day with a recommended cream or lotion.
- Protect from the sun using a sunblock with an SPF 15 or higher.
- Protect from irritations that can be caused by:
  - *chemicals* such as cleaning solutions or solvents
  - *mechanical irritation* such as continuous rubbing of belts or tight clothing
  - *physical irritation* such as extreme heat and cold, or cuts and scrapes

---

TIP If the patient is still undergoing radiation treatment, it is important to use products that will not interfere with radiation therapy.

BIBLIOGRAPHY

Cooper, D. 1992. Acute surgical wounds. In *Acute and chronic wounds*, ed. R. Bryant, 91–100. St. Louis, MO: Mosby-Year Book.

Kane, D. 1997. Surgical repair. In *Chronic wound care: A clinical source book for health care professionals*, 2d ed., eds. D. Krasner and D. Kane, 235–244. Wayne, PA: Health Management Publications.

Medelsohn, F. A. et al. 2002. Wound care after radiation therapy. *Advances in Skin & Wound Care* 15(5), 216–224.

Mulder, D. et al. 1998. *Clinicians pocket guide to chronic wound repair.* Springhouse, PA: Springhouse Corporation.

Porock, D., et al. 1999. Management of radiation skin reactions: Literature review and clinical application. *Plastic Surgical Nursing* 19(4), 185–192.

Wysocki, A., and Bryant R. 1992. Skin. In *Acute and chronic wounds: Nursing management*, ed. R. Bryant. 1–25. St. Louis, MO: Mosby-Year Book.

PART IV

Issues Specific to Home Health and Skilled Nursing Facilities

CHAPTER 13

Documentation and Compliance in Home Health Care

Ben Peirce

Documentation requirements for certified home health care agencies are largely determined by the Centers for Medicare and Medicaid Services (CMS) regulations and billing requirements. Home health care for patients with commercial insurance is organized differently. A case manager approves visits on a weekly basis. These case managers, however, usually expect the same information that CMS now requires to approve visits.

In 2000, the CMS regulations changed from payment on a fee for service basis to a prospective payment system. This change had a profound impact on how home health is organized.

Trends in wound care in the home include:

- focus on objective wound assessment and documentation to measure progress
- use of protocols or pathways with timeframes to guide visit activities
- use of follow-up case conferences periodically to reevaluate care

Since October of 2000, payment for services by CMS is based on the Outcome and Assessment Information Set (OASIS) data collected at the start of home health care, resumption of care, and discharge. Payment covers two months of service regardless of how many visits or what type of supplies are provided. The amount a home care agency receives varies significantly depending on the patient's clinical condition, functional level, and the use of therapy services.

The OASIS dataset is generated from the assessment done by the admitting nurse or therapist using a standardized set of questions and must be supported by other assessment information collected at the same time. Together, these two components form the initial skilled assessment that is the basis of the home health plan of care, also known as the HCFA Form 485. This information must be transmitted electronically to CMS on admission and discharge in order to be paid for services. Because all reimbursement is based on this OASIS assessment data, clinicians and their managers now understand that effective assessment is critical to successful home health care. In addition to using OASIS as the basis for payment, CMS is also comparing patient condition at discharge to condition at admission to identify OASIS-related patient outcomes and is instructing state and federal surveyors to use the data to help guide the survey process.

Twenty-two of the OASIS assessment questions affect payment, and four of these are based on the assessment of wounds. Data from these questions are also being analyzed by CMS to measure patient outcomes to help inform the public about the quality of care as they select possible providers and to guide state and federal surveys. It is therefore important to understand how to answer these questions accurately and consistently.

M0230 and M0240 are the primary and secondary diagnoses. Diagnoses in five categories affect reimbursement: neurologic, orthopedic, diabetic, traumatic, and burns (if associated with a wound). Clinicians should use care to ensure that these are selected appropriately. If omitted, earned revenue is lost and if added incorrectly, the agency could lose the revenue later on a retrospective review by Medicare.

- M0230   Primary Diagnosis (_____)   +   Severity Rating____
- M0240   Other Diagnosis (_____)   +   Severity Rating____

Severity Rating
- 0—Asymptomatic, no treatment needed at this time
- 1—Symptoms well controlled with current therapy
- 2—Symptoms controlled with difficulty, affecting daily functioning; patient needs ongoing monitoring
- 3—Symptoms poorly controlled, patient needs frequent adjustment in treatment and dose monitoring
- 4—Symptoms poorly controlled, history of rehospitalizations

Early feedback from clinicians to CMS suggested that the OASIS questions on wound status were difficult to answer because the terminology lacked universal definitions (fully granulating, early/partial granulation, nonhealing). In response to these issues, the WOCN Society identified and validated definitions in the OASIS Guidance document (see page 221) that was accepted by CMS as appropriate for use when answering OASIS questions. The OASIS Guidance document can be a valuable addition to OASIS training tools for home health agencies.

WOCN GUIDANCE ON OASIS SKIN AND WOUND STATUS M0 ITEMS

Overview and Background

As mandated by the Balanced Budget Act of 1997, Home Health Reimbursement shifted to a prospective payment system effective October 2000. Under this system, payment is based on the patient's clinical severity, functional status, and therapy requirements. The system for wound classification uses terms such as "nonhealing," and "partially granulating," and "fully granulating"; these terms lack universal definition and clinicians have verbalized concerns that they may be interpreting these terms incorrectly. The WOCN Society has therefore developed the following guidelines for classification of wounds. These items were developed by consensus among the WOCN's panel of content experts.

M0 445: Does the patient have a Pressure Ulcer?

M0 450: Current number of Pressure Ulcers at Each Stage

M0 460: Stage of Most Problematic (Observable) Pressure Ulcer

    1   Stage I

    2   Stage II

    3   Stage III

    4   Stage IV

   NA No observable pressure ulcer

Definitions

Pressure Ulcer: Any lesion caused by unrelieved pressure resulting in damage of underlying tissue. Pressure ulcers are usually located over bony prominences and are staged to classify the degree of tissue damage observed.

    Stage I: Non-blanchable erythema of intact skin, the heralding lesion of skin ulceration. In individuals with darker skin, discoloration of the skin, warmth, edema, induration, or hardness may also be indicators.

    Stage II: Partial thickness skin loss involving epidermis, dermis, or both. The ulcer is superficial and presents as an abrasion, blister, or shallow crater.

    Stage III: Full thickness skin loss involving damage to or necrosis of subcutaneous tissue that may extend down to, but not through, underlying fascia. The ulcer presents clinically as a deep crater with or without undermining of adjacent tissue.

    Stage IV: Full thickness skin loss with extensive destruction, tissue necrosis, or damage to muscle, bone, or supporting structures (e.g., tendon, joint capsule). Undermining and sinus tracts may also be associated with Stage IV pressure ulcers.

Non-observable: Wound is unable to be visualized due to an orthopedic device, dressing, etc. A pressure ulcer cannot be accurately staged until the deepest viable tissue layer is visible; this means that wounds covered with eschar and/or slough cannot be staged, and should be documented as non-observable.

M0 464: Status of Most Problematic (Observable) Pressure Ulcer

    1   Fully granulating

    2   Early/partial granulation

    3   Not healing

    NA No observable pressure ulcer

- **Fully Granulating:** Wound bed filled with granulation tissue to the level of the surrounding skin or new epithelium; no dead space, no avascular tissue; no signs or symptoms of infection; wound edges are open.

- **Early/Partial Granulation:** >25% of the wound bed is covered with granulation tissue; there is minimal avascular tissue (i.e., <25% of the wound bed is covered with avascular tissue); may have dead space; no signs or symptoms of infection; wound edges open.

- **Non-healing:** Wound with >25% avascular tissue OR signs/symptoms of infection OR clean but non-granulating wound bed OR closed/hyperkeratotic wound edges OR persistent failure to improve despite appropriate comprehensive wound management. Note: a new Stage 1 pressure ulcer is reported on OASIS as not healing.

M0 468: Does the patient have a stasis ulcer?

M0 470: Current number of Observable Stasis Ulcer(s)

M0 474: Does this patient have at least one Stasis Ulcer that cannot be observed?

M0 476: Status of the Most Problematic (Observable) Stasis Ulcer

    1   Fully granulating

    2   Early/partial granulation

    3   Not healing

    NA No observable stasis ulcer

Definitions

Fully Granulating: Wound bed filled with granulation tissue to the level of the surrounding skin or new epithelium; no dead space, no avascular tissue; no signs or symptoms of infection; wound edges are open.

Early/Partial Granulation: > 25% of the wound bed is covered with granulation tissue; there is minimal avascular tissue (i.e., <25% of the wound bed is covered with avascular tissue); may have dead space; no signs or symptoms of infection; wound edges open.

Non-healing: Wound with >25% avascular tissue OR signs/symptoms of infection OR clean but non-granulating wound bed OR closed/hyperkeratotic wound edges OR persistent failure to improve despite appropriate comprehensive wound management.

M0 482: Does the patient have a Surgical Wound?

M0 484: Current number of (Observable) Surgical Wounds

M0 486: Does the patient have at least one Surgical Wound that cannot be observed due to the presence of a non-removable dressing?

M0 488: Status of the most problematic (Observable) Surgical Wound

     1   Fully granulating

     2   Early/partial granulation

     3   Not healing

     NA No observable surgical wound

Description/Classification of Wounds Healing by Primary Intention
(i.e., approximated incisions)

- Fully granulating/healing: incision well-approximated with complete epithelialization of incision; no signs or symptoms of infection; healing ridge well defined

- Early/partial granulation: incision well-approximated but not completely epithelialized; no signs or symptoms of infection; healing ridge palpable but poorly defined

- Non-healing: incisional separation OR incisional necrosis OR signs or symptoms of infection OR no palpable healing ridge

Description/Classification of Wounds Healing by Secondary Intention
(i.e., healing of dehisced wound by granulation, contraction, and epithelialization)

- **Fully Granulating:** Wound bed filled with granulation tissue to the level of the surrounding skin or new epithelium; no dead space, no avascular tissue; no signs or symptoms of infection; wound edges are open.

- **Early/Partial Granulation:** > 25% of the wound bed is covered with granulation tissue; there is minimal avascular tissue (i.e., <25% of the wound bed is covered with avascular tissue); may have dead space; no signs or symptoms of infection; wound edges are open.

- **Non-healing:** Wound with > 25% avascular tissue OR signs/symptoms of infection OR clean but non-granulating wound bed OR closed/hyperkeratotic wound edges OR persistent failure to improve despite comprehensive appropriate wound management.

Glossary

Avascular: Lacking in blood supply; synonyms are dead, devitalized, necrotic, and nonviable. Specific types include slough and eschar.

Clean Wound: Wound free of devitalized tissue, purulent drainage, foreign material or debris

Closed Wound Edges: Edges of top layers of epidermis have rolled down to cover lower edge of epidermis, including basement membrane, so that epithelial cells cannot migrate from wound edges; also described as epibole. Presents clinically as sealed edge of mature epithelium; may be hard/thickened; may be discolored (i.e., yellowish, gray, or white).

Dead Space: A defect or cavity

Dehisced/Dehiscence: Separation of surgical incision; loss of approximation of wound edges

Epidermis: Outermost layer of skin

Epithelialization: Regeneration of epidermis across a wound surface

Eschar: Black or brown necrotic, devitalized tissue; tissue can be loose or firmly adherent, hard, soft or soggy.

Full Thickness: Tissue damage involving total loss of epidermis and dermis and extending into the subcutaneous tissue and possibly into the muscle or bone

Granulation Tissue: The pink/red, moist tissue comprised of new blood vessels, connective tissue, fibroblasts, and inflammatory cells, which fills an open wound when it starts to heal; typically appears deep pink or red with an irregular, "berry-like" surface

Healing: A dynamic process involving synthesis of new tissue for repair of skin and soft tissue defects.

Healing Ridge: Palpatory finding indicative of new collagen synthesis. Palpation reveals induration beneath the skin that extends to approximately 1 cm on each side of the wound. Becomes evident between 5 and 9 days after wounding; typically persists till about 15 days post-wounding. This is an expected positive sign.

Hyperkeratosis: Hard, white/gray tissue surrounding the wound

Infection: The presence of bacteria or other microorganisms in sufficient quantity to damage tissue or impair healing. Wounds can be classified as infected when the wound tissue contains 10^5 (100,000) or greater microorganisms per gram of tissue. Typical signs and symptoms of infection include purulent exudate, odor, erythema, warmth, tenderness, edema, pain, fever, and elevated white cell count. However, clinical signs of infection may not be present, especially in the immunocompromised patient or the patient with poor perfusion.

Necrotic Tissue: See *Avascular.*

Non-granulating: Absence of granulation tissue; wound surface appears smooth as opposed to granular. For example, in a wound that is clean but non-granulating, the wound surface appears smooth and red as opposed to berry-like.

Partial Thickness: Confined to the skin layers; damage does not penetrate below the dermis and may be limited to the epidermal layers only

Sinus Tract: Course or path of tissue destruction occurring in any direction from the surface or edge of the wound; results in dead space with potential for abscess formation. Also sometimes called "tunneling." (Can be distinguished from undermining by fact that the sinus tract involves a small portion of the wound edge whereas undermining involves a significant portion of the wound edge.)

Slough: Soft moist avascular (devitalized) tissue; may be white, yellow, tan, or green; may be loose or firmly adherent

Tunnelinor: See *Sinus Tract*

Undermining: Area of tissue destruction extending under intact skin along the periphery of a wound; commonly seen in shear injuries. Can be distinguished from sinus tract by the fact that undermining involves a significant portion of the wound edge, whereas sinus tract involves only a small portion of the wound edge.

In addition to being skilled at OASIS assessments, clinicians must also be skilled at describing wounds in a narrative note or on wound assessment forms because the OASIS dataset alone is not adequate to meet the requirements for a skilled assessment in a certified home health agency.

In terms of assessing wounds, validated tools are not currently available though progress has been made in this area. The following physical characteristics are emerging as key components of a complete wound assessment, and should be documented initially and regularly thereafter. These include wound location, size, tissue type, and exudate amount. Wound assessments should also be documented with any significant change in condition, such as after a significant debridement, with increasing pain, or signs of infection. (Wound assessment is covered in detail in Chapter 2.)

For patients with common conditions, evidence-based pathways or protocols should be used as the starting point for individualizing the plan of care. These pathways should include specific activities and time frames to ensure each home health visit progresses the patient and family closer to the goal of stability and a maximum level of independence. Documentation should also note case conferences with regular reviews of progress and discussions of modifying the plan of care, as needed. This helps maintain a realistic plan with achievable goals for the individual patient.

Objective wound assessment should be an integral part of the regular system assessment clinicians perform and should be consistent with the OASIS dataset. When documented well, they support care that is ethically sound, reimbursable, and compliant with state and federal regulations.

BIBLIOGRAPHY

Bates, Jensen et al. 1992. Validity and reliability of the pressure sore status tool. *Decubitus* (5)6, 20–28.

CMS's Home Health Care Quality Initiative, http://www.cms.hhs.gov/quality/hhqi, April 2004.

CMS's OASIS Overview, http://www.cms.hhs.qov/oasis/hhoview.asp, April 2004.

Leslie, Cheryl M. 2003. The changes impacting wound care practices. *The Remington Report* 11(3), 14–17.

WOCN Society OASIS Guidance Document, www.wocn.orq, April 2004.

Zuber R. 2003. Medicare survey shifts focus to outcomes. *Home Healthcare Nurse* (21)3, 187-191.

CHAPTER 14

Documentation and Compliance in Skilled Nursing Facilities

Susan V. McGovern

Patients requiring continued wound care following hospitalization may need a higher level of skilled care than can be provided at home by either the patient and/or family/support system, or by visits from a home health service provider. Federally funded skilled nursing facilities (SNFs) have specific regulations that must be followed related to admission criteria, resident assessments and documentation, and types of services provided.

A skilled service is defined as a service provided where the inherent complexity of that service is such that it can be safely and effectively performed only by or under the general supervision of skilled nursing or skilled rehabilitation personnel. Examples of skilled services, in addition to direct skilled nursing services, include

- management and evaluation of a Patient Care Plan
- observation and assessment of a patient's condition
- teaching and training activities

Care in an SNF is covered if all the following are true:

1. The patient requires skilled nursing services or skilled rehabilitation services (i.e., services that must be performed by or under the supervision of a professional or technical person).
2. The patient requires the skilled services on a daily basis.
3. The daily skilled services can be provided only on an inpatient basis in an SNF.

If any one of these three factors is not met, a stay in an SNF is not covered. If the above three factors are met, for those clients covered by Medicare, post-hospital extended care services for inpatient SNF services are covered under Part A. The admission criteria for SNFs are as follows:

- The beneficiary must have had an inpatient hospitalization for a medically necessary stay of at least 3 consecutive calendar days.
- The patient must also have been transferred to the SNF within 30 days after discharge from the hospital. (Exceptions are defined in the Health Care Financing Administration [HCFA] "Skilled Nursing Facility Manual".)
- The services to be provided must be needed for a condition that was treated during the patient's hospital stay, or for a condition that arose while the patient was in the hospital.

A beneficiary is eligible for 100 days of care in an SNF during the benefit period. (See HCFA "Skilled Nursing Facility Manual" for more detailed criteria and exemptions.)

A federal reform law, the Balanced Budget Act of 1997 (BBA 1997), contained major changes related to reimbursement in all health care facilities. The BBA 1997 converted the previous SNF cost-based reimbursement system, Medicare Part A, to a prospective payment system (PPS). This PPS bundles all routine, ancillary, and capital costs into a single per diem payment to the SNF based on patient acuity. The SNF admission criteria, as defined above, remain the same under this system.

Coverage determinations, or level of care determinations, have been simplified by a system for classifying residents based on resource utilization known as Resource Utilization Groups, Version III (RUG-III). Facilities will utilize information obtained from the Minimum Data Set, Version 2 (MDS), an assessment tool; and the Resident Assessment Instrument (RAI) to classify residents into RUG-III groups. For Medicare billing purposes there is a payment code for each of the RUG-III groups, so it is imperative to appropriately assess each individual to receive adequate payment for services provided.

The RAI was developed following the Omnibus Budget Reconciliation Act of 1987 (OBRA 1987), which contained nursing home reform laws. OBRA 1987 was implemented by the federal government to improve clinical care and outcomes in skilled nursing facilities by providing a regulatory framework that required a standardized approach to the assessment of residents in SNFs. Federally funded SNFs use the RAI to identify a resident's strengths and needs, which are then addressed in an individualized care plan.

The RAI consists of three components:

1. The Minimum Data Set, Version 2 (MDS)—a set of screening, clinical, and functional status elements that form the basis of the com-

prehensive assessment for all residents of long-term care facilities certified to participate in the Medicare/Medicaid program.

2. Resident Assessment Protocols (RAPs)—a component of the utilization guidelines. The RAPs are a framework for organizing MDS information and examining additional clinically relevant information about the resident. RAPs help identify social, medical, and psychological problems for which an individualized care plan can then be developed. They are triggered by specific components on the MDS.

3. Utilization Guidelines—instructions concerning when and how to use the RAI.

An RAI must be completed on any individual residing more than 14 days on a unit of a facility that is certified as a long-term care facility for participants in the Medicare or Medicaid program. Comprehensive RAI assessments require completion of the MDS, a review of the triggered RAPs, and review of the comprehensive Care Plan. Care Plan development must be completed within 7 days of the MDS completion. The time frame for completion of the MDS assessment, according to OBRA 1987 and the Medicare PPS mandates of the BBA 1997, is as follows:

- Admission assessment—completed initially by the 5th day of a resident's stay and a full assessment by the 14th day. The assessment must then be updated on the 30th, 60th, and 90th day of a resident's stay.
- Annual reassessment—completed within 12 months of the most recent full assessment
- Significant change in status reassessment—completed by the end of the 14th calendar day following a significant change in the resident's condition. A significant change is defined as a major change in the resident's status that
  - is not self-limiting (for example, catching the flu or a cold)
  - affects on more than one area of the resident's health status
  - requires an interdisciplinary review or revision of the Care Plan
- Quarterly assessment—a set of MDS items, mandated by federal and state regulations, that must be completed no less frequently than every 3 months

The MDS contains a section specific to skin and wound conditions, Section M: Skin Condition (Exhibit 14–1, page 231). Ulcers, pressure, and stasis that have been identified within 7 days of the assessment are documented and staged. Additional skin and foot problems are also included on the MDS. Skin treatment, including pressure-relieving devices, turning programs, nutrition, and hydration interventions, should be listed. The presence of ulcers, in addition to other risk factors, such as bed mobility problems, bladder and bowel incontinence, peripheral vascular disease, and diabetes mellitus, identified on the MDS will trigger the Pressure Ulcer RAP (Exhibit 14–2, page 233). It is important to include on the MDS all factors that influence the resident's current health care status. This will have a direct correlation on the RUG-III category assigned and the reimbursement for care paid to the SNFs.

The Care Plan will be developed by a review of the MDS, the triggered RAPs, and other identified issues or problems that will influence the resident's health status outcome, and should include current nutrition and hydration status. The resident's individual needs should also be included in the Care Plan. For example, a resident with a diabetic foot ulcer may have poor compliance with following a specific diet. This should be identified in the Care Plan along with potential interventions, such as a consult with the dietitian for ongoing dietary teaching with the resident and spouse/care-giver. Discharge planning should be identified on admission, be included as part of the resident's Care Plan, and be discussed at each interdisciplinary team meeting.

The following points are important to keep in mind when caring for residents with wounds and documenting in their medical record:

- A complete assessment and note detailing the assessment of the wound should be included in the admission process.
- A skin risk assessment is an integral part of the admission assessment. Standardized tools, such as the Braden Scale for Predicting Pressure Sore Risk (Exhibit 6–2, page 102) may be used.
- The physician's order for wound care should be reviewed, and if the care ordered is not appropriate to the status of the wound, the physician needs to be contacted and a new order obtained.
- A complete assessment of the wound, including measurements (length, width, depth, and stage), should be documented at least weekly. Reverse staging is not acceptable since the tissue that fills in the wound is granulation/scar tissue and is not the same as the original skin or muscle.
- Implementation of Care Plan interventions and an evaluation of the resident's response to the interventions should be included in the progress notes.

Exhibit 14–1 MDS Section M: Skin Condition

1.	**ULCERS (Due to any cause)**	*(Record the number of ulcers at each ulcer stage—regardless of cause. If none present at a stage, record "0" (zero).* **Code all that apply during last 7 days. Code 9 = 9 or more.)** **[Requires full body exam.]**	**Number at Stage**
		a. **Stage 1.** A persistent area of skin redness (with- out a break in the skin) that does not disappear when pressure is relieved.	■
		b. **Stage 2.** A partial thickness loss of skin lay-ers that presents clinically as an abrasion, blister, or shallow crater.	■
		c. **Stage 3.** A full thickness of skin is lost, exposing the subcutaneous tis-sues—presents as a deep crater with or with-out undermining adjacent tissue.	■
		d. **Stage 4.** A full thickness of skin and subcu-taneous tissue is lost, exposing muscle or bone.	■
2.	**TYPE OF ULCER**	*(For each type of ulcer,* **code for the highest stage in the last 7 days** *using scale in item M1: 0 = none; stages 1, 2, 3, 4)*	
		a. Pressure ulcer—any lesion caused by pres-sure resulting in damage of underlying tis-sue 1 = 16; 2, 3, or 4 = 12, 16	■
		b. Stasis ulcer—open lesion caused by poor circulation in the lower extremities	■
3.	**HISTORY OF RESOLVED ULCERS**	Resident had an ulcer that was resolved or cured in **LAST 90 DAYS** 0. No 1. Yes 16	■
4.	**OTHER SKIN PROB-LEMS OR LESIONS PRESENT**	**(Check all that apply** *during* **last 7 days)** Abrasions, bruises Burns (second or third degree) Open lesions other than ulcers, rashes, cuts (e.g., cancer lesions) Rashes (e.g., intertrigo, eczema, drug rash, heat rash, herpes zoster)	a. b. c. d.

continues

Exhibit 14–1 continued

	OTHER SKIN PROB-LEMS OR LESIONS PRESENT (continued)	Skin desnsitized to pain or pressure	e.
		Skin tears or cuts (other than surgery)	f.
		Surgical wounds	g.
		NONE OF ABOVE	h.
5.	**SKIN TREATMENTS**	***(Check all that apply*** *during* **last 7 days)**	
		Pressure relieving device(s) for chair	a.
		Pressure relieving device(s) for bed	b.
		Turning/repositioning program	c.
		Nutrition or hydration intervention to manage skin problems	d.
		Ulcer care	e.
		Surgical wound care	f.
		Application of dressings (with or without topical medications) other than to feet	g.
		Application of ointments/medications (other than to feet)	h.
		Other preventative or protective skin care (other than to feet)	i.
		NONE OF ABOVE	j.
6.	**FOOT PROBLEMS AND CARE**	***(Check all that apply*** *during* **last 7 days)**	
		Resident has one or more foot problems (e.g., corns, calluses, bunions, hammer toes, overlapping toes, pain, structural problems)	a.
		Infection of the foot (e.g., cellulitis, purulent drainage)	b.
		Open lesions on the foot	c.
		Nails/calluses trimmed during **last 90 days**	d.
		Received preventative or protective foot care (e.g., used special shoes, inserts, pads, toe separators)	e.
		Application of dressings (with or without topical medications)	f.
		NONE OF ABOVE	g.

Exhibit 14–2 Resident Assessment Protocol: Pressure Ulcers

PzLEM

Between 3 percent and 5 percent (or more) of residents in nursing facilities have pressure ulcers (pressure sores, decubitus ulcers, bedsores). Sixty percent or more of residents will typically be at risk of pressure ulcer development. Pressure ulcers can have serious consequences for the elderly and are costly and time-consuming to treat. However, they are one of the most common, preventable, and treatable conditions among the elderly who have restricted mobility. Successful outcomes can be expected with preventive and treatment programs.

Assessment goals are (1) to ensure that a treatment plan is in place for residents with pressure ulcers, and (2) to identify residents at risk for developing a pressure ulcer who are not currently receiving some type of preventive care program.

TRIGGERS

Pressure ulcer present or there is a risk for occurrence if one or more of following present (risk):

- pressure Ulcer(s) Present (present)[a]
  [M2a = 1,2,3,4]
- bed mobility problem (risk)
  [G1aA = 2,3,4,8][b]
- bedfast (risk)
  [G6a = checked]
- bowel incontinence (risk)
  [H1a = 1,2,3,4]
- peripheral vascular disease (risk)
  [I1j = checked]
- previous pressure ulcer (risk)
  [M3 = 1]
- skin desensitized to pain or pressure (risk)
  [M4e = checked]
- daily Trunk Restraint (risk)[c]
  [P4c = 2]

(a) Note: Codes 2, 3, and 4 also trigger on the Nutritional Status RAP.
(b) Note: Codes 2, 3, and 4 also trigger on the ADL RAP.
(c) Note: This code also triggers on the Falls RAP and Physical Restraints RAP.

continues

Exhibit 14–2 continued

GUIDELINES

Review the MDS items listed on the RAP key for relevance in understanding the type of care that may be required.

Diagnoses, Conditions, and Treatments that Present Complications

Consider carefully whether the resident exhibits conditions or is receiving treatments that may either place the resident at higher risk of developing pressure ulcers or complicate the treatment. Such conditions include:

- diabetes, Alzheimer's disease, and other dementias. An impairment in cognitive ability, particularly severe end-stage dementia, can lead to immobility.

- edema. The presence of extravascular fluid can impair blood flow. If prolonged or excess pressure is applied to an area with edema, skin breakdown can occur.

- antidepressants and antianxiety/hypnotics. These medications can produce or contribute to lessened mobility, worsen incontinence, and lead to or increase confusion.

Interventions/Programs to Consider If the Resident Develops a New Pressure Ulcer, or an Ulcer Being Treated Is Not Resolved

A variety of factors may explain this occurrence; however, they may suggest the need to evaluate current interventions and modifications of the care plan.

- Review the resident's medical condition, medications, and other risk factors to determine whether the care plan (for prevention or cure) addresses all potential causes or complications.

- Review the care plan to determine whether it is actually being followed (e.g., is the resident being turned often enough to prevent ulcer formation).

Things to Consider If The Resident Is at Risk for Pressure Ulcers but Is Not Receiving Preventive Skin Care

Even if pressure ulcers are not present, determine why this course of prevention is not being provided to a resident with risk factors.

- Is the resident new to the unit?

- Do few or many risk factors for the development of pressure ulcers apply to this resident?

- Are staff concentrating on other problems (e.g., resolution of behavior problems) so that the risks of pressure ulcers are masked?

continues

Exhibit 14–2 continued

PRESSURE ULCERS RAP KEY (FOR MDS VERSION 2.0)

Trigger—Revision

Pressure ulcer present or risk for occurrence if one or more of following present:

- Pressure ulcer(s) present (Present)[a] [M2a = 1,2,3,4]

- Bed mobility problem (Risk) [G1aA = 2,3,4,8][b]

- Bedfast (Risk) [G6a = checked]

- Bowel incontinence (Risk) [H1a = 1,2,3,4]

- Peripheral vascular disease (Risk) [I1j = checked]

- Previous ulcer (Risk) [M3 =1]

- Skin desensitized to pain or pressure (Risk) [M4e = checked]

- Daily trunk restraint (Risk)[c] [P4c = 2]

Guidelines

Other factors that address or may complicate treatment of pressure ulcers or risk of ulcers:

- Diagnoses or conditions: Diabetes [I1a], Alzheimer's disease [I1q], Other dementia [I1u], Hemiplegia/Hemiparesis [I1v], Multiple Sclerosis [I1w], Edema [J1g]

- Interventions/Programs:

  - Pressure relieving chair/beds [M5a, M5b]

  - Turning/repositioning [M5c]

  - Nutrition or hydration program to manage skin care problems [M5d]

  - Ulcer care [M5e]

  - Surgical wound care/treatment [M5f]

  - Application of dressings (with or with- out topical medications) other than to feet [M5g]

  - Application of ointment/medications (other than to feet) [M5h]

  - Preventive or protective skin care (other than to feet) [M5i]

  - Preventive or protective foot care [M6e]

  - Application of dressings to feet (with or without topical medications) [M6f]

  - Use of restraints [P4c,d,e]

- Medications:

  Antipsychotics [O4a]

  Antianxiety [O4b]

  Antidepressants [O4c]

  Hypnotics [O4d]

[a]Note: Codes 2, 3, and 4 also trigger on the Nutritional Status RAP.
[b]Note: Codes 2, 3, and 4 also trigger on the ADL RAP.
[c]Note: This code also triggers on the Falls RAP and Physical Restraints RAP.

- Documentation should reflect when each dressing change was performed, any teaching provided, and the resident's response to the care provided. Any change in the wound noted at the time of the dressing change must be reflected in the note (for example, there is less drainage and inflammation than previously, or perhaps there is an increase in drainage and an odor is now present).
- HCFA mandates that the MDS be updated if there are significant changes in the resident's status. A healing wound, although it might be considered a significant change, does not trigger the need for an update due to the fact that this is the planned goal of treatment. If a clean, healing wound deteriorates, for example, and now has purulent, foul-smelling drainage and increased erythema and the resident develops pain at the site, spikes a fever, and becomes confused, this change would require a review and update of the MDS and Care Plan. The physician must be notified and the changes reported so appropriate orders may be obtained.
- Nonhealing wounds provide a particular challenge to clinicians. If a wound has not progressed toward healing within 2 weeks of a specific treatment, the physician should be notified and a different wound care protocol considered. This is an excellent time for the wound care team to evaluate the wound and make a recommendation for another type of treatment.

Many facilities have specific wound care forms for documentation. It is helpful to document the wound assessment and care in one consistent place in the medical record. It is very difficult to monitor the progress of a wound if the first assessment is on the Skin/Wound Flowsheet and the next assessment is documented in the progress notes. Be sure to follow your facility's policies related to wound care assessment and documentation.

Effective documentation is essential in SNFs. It will demonstrate a resident's progress or lack of progress (and reasons why) toward an identified outcome, it will reflect the quality of the care provided, and finally, it will have a direct impact on reimbursement for care provided by the facility.

BIBLIOGRAPHY

Health Care Financing Administration. "Skilled Nursing Facility Manual." On line. Internet. 8 March 2000. http://www.hcfa.gov/pubforms/12_SNF/sn00.htm

Health Care Financing Administration. "SNF Prospective Payment System." On line. Internet. 8 March 2000. http://www.hcfa.gov/medicare/snfpps.htm

Health Care Financing Administration's Minimum Data Set, Resident Assessment Protocols, and Utilization Guidelines, version 2.0. 1995. In *Long term care facility resident assessment instrument (RAI) user's manual. Life Sciences Network of Illinois.*

Abscess. A circumscribed collection of pus that forms in tissue as a result of acute or chronic localized infection. It is associated with tissue destruction and frequently swelling.

Acute Wounds. Disruptions in the skin integrity and underlying tissues that progress through the healing process in a timely manner without complications.

Adherent Materials. Matter attached to the wound bed such as eschar, dirt particles, or bacteria.

Albumin. A major plasma protein. Numerous studies have revealed increased morbidity and mortality in patients with decreased serum albumin levels. The normal serum albumin concentration is 3.5 to 5.0 gm/dL. This value is effective showing nutritional status 3–4 weeks prior to lab draw. (See *Hypoalbuminemia*)

Ankle-Brachial Index. Doppler-derived lower extremity arterial pressures are measured and an ankle-brachial index (ABI) is calculated by making a ratio of pressure at the ankle to pressure in the arm. The normal ABI is 0.9 to 1.1.

Antiseptic (Topical). Product with antimicrobial activity designed for use on skin or other superficial tissues; may damage cells.

Arterial Ulcer. Wounds that are caused by insufficient arterial perfusion. These wounds are usually painful. Clinically, they may appear as "punched out" wounds that have pale wound beds, well-defined wound edges, and minimal exudate.

Atherosclerosis. Plaque formation on the walls of arteries causing a narrowing of the lumen and decreased blood flow.

Bottoming Out. Expression used to describe inadequate support from a mattress overlay or seat cushion as determined by a "hand check." To perform a hand check, the caregiver places an outstretched hand (palm up) under the overlay or cushion below the pressure ulcer or that part of the body at risk for a pressure ulcer. If the caregiver feels less than an inch of support material, the patient has bottomed out and the support surface is therefore inadequate.

Cellulitis. Inflammation of cellular or connective tissue. Inflammation may be diminished or absent in immunosuppressed individuals.

Cellulitis (Advancing). Cellulitis that is visibly spreading in the area of the wound. Advancement can be monitored by marking the outer edge of the cellulitis and assessing the area for advancement or spread 24 hours later.

Chronic Wounds. These nonhealing wounds deviate from the expected sequence of repair in terms of time, appearance, and response to appropriate treatments.

Clean. Containing no foreign material or debris.

Clean Dressing. Dressing that is not sterile but is free of environmental contaminants such as water damage, dust, pest and rodent contaminants, and gross soiling.

Clean Wound. Wound free of purulent drainage, devitalized tissue, or dirt.

Colonized. The presence of bacteria on the surface or in the tissue of a wound without indications of infection such as purulent exudate, foul odor, or surrounding inflammation. All Stage II, III, and IV pressure ulcers are colonized.

Contaminated. Containing bacteria, other microorganisms, or foreign material. The term usually refers to bacterial contamination and in this context is synonymous with colonized. Wounds with bacterial counts of 10^5 organisms per gram of tissue or less are generally considered contaminated; those with higher counts are generally considered infected.

Culture and Sensitivity. Removal of bacteria from a wound for the purpose of placing them in a growth medium in the laboratory to propagate to the point where they can be identified and tested for sensitivity to various antibiotics.

Culture (Swab). Technique involving the use of a swab to remove bacteria from a wound and place them in a growth medium for propagation and identification. Swab cultures obtained from the surface of a pressure ulcer are usually positive because of surface colonization and should not be used to diagnose ulcer infection.

Dead Space. A cavity remaining in a wound.

Debridement. Removal of devitalized tissue and foreign matter from a wound. Various methods can be used for this purpose:

Autolytic Debridement. The use of synthetic dressings to cover a wound and allow eschar to self-digest by the action of enzymes present in wound fluids.

Enzymatic (Chemical) Debridement. The topical application of pro-teolytic substances (enzymes) to break down devitalized tissue.

Mechanical Debridement. Removal of foreign material and devital-ized or contaminated tissue from a wound by physical forces rather than by chemical (enzymatic) or natural (autolytic) forces. Examples are wet-to-dry dressings, wound irrigation, whirlpool, and dextranomers.

Sharp Debridement. Removal of foreign material or devitalized tis-sue by a sharp instrument such as a scalpel. Laser debridement is also considered a type of sharp debridement.

Dehiscence. Separation of the layers of a surgical wound.

Dermis. Inner layer of skin that contains the hair follicles and sweat glands. A stage II pressure ulcer will involve this layer of skin.

Deterioration. Negative course. Failure of the pressure ulcer to heal, as shown by wound enlargement that is not brought about by debride-ment.

Dextranomers. Highly hydrophilic dextran-polymer beads that are poured into secreting wounds to absorb wound exudates and act as a debriding agent.

Dressing. The material applied to a wound for the protection of the wound and absorbance of drainage.

Alginate Dressing. A nonwoven, absorptive dressing manufactured from seaweed.

Film Dressing. A clear, adherent, nonabsorptive, polymer-based dressing that is permeable to oxygen and water vapor but not to water.

Foam Dressing. A spongelike polymer dressing that may or may not be adherent; it may be impregnated or coated with other materi-als and has some absorptive properties.

Gauze Dressing. A cotton or synthetic fabric dressing that is absorp-tive and permeable to water, water vapor, and oxygen. This dress-ing may be impregnated with petrolatum, antiseptics, or other agents.

Continuously Moist Saline Gauze. A dressing technique in which gauze moistened with normal saline is applied to the wound and remoistened frequently enough so it will remain moist. The goal is to maintain a continuously moist wound environment.

Wet-to-Dry Saline Gauze. A dressing technique in which gauze moistened with normal saline is applied wet to the wound and removed once the gauze becomes dry and adheres to the wound bed. The goal is to debride the wound as the dressing is removed.

Hydrocolloid Dressing. An adhesive, moldable wafer made of a carbohydrate-based material, usually with a waterproof backing. This dressing usually is impermeable to oxygen, water, and water vapor and has some absorptive properties.

Hydrogel Dressing. A water-based, nonadherent, polymer-based dressing that has some absorptive properties.

Pastes/Powders/Beads. Agents formulated primarily to fill wound cavities that may have some absorptive properties.

Epidermis. Avascular outer layer of the skin.

Epithelialization. The stage of tissue healing in which the epithelial cells migrate (move) across the surface of a wound. During this stage of healing, the epithelium appears the color of "ground glass" to pink.

Erythema. Redness of the skin.

Blanchable Erythema. Reddened area that temporarily turns white or pale when pressure is applied with a fingertip. Blanchable erythema over a pressure site is usually due to a normal reactive hyperemic response.

Nonblanchable Erythema. Redness that persists when fingertip pressure is applied. Nonblanchable erythema over a pressure site is a symptom of a Stage I pressure ulcer.

Eschar. Thick, leathery, necrotic, devitalized tissue.

Exudate. Any fluid that has been extruded from a tissue or its capillaries, more specifically because of injury or inflammation. It is characteristically high in protein and white blood cells.

Fascia. A sheet or band of fibrous tissue that lies deep below the skin or encloses muscles and various organs of the body.

Fluid Irrigation. Cleansing by means of a stream of fluid, preferably saline.

Friction. Mechanical force exerted when skin is dragged across a coarse surface such as bed linens.

Full-Thickness Tissue Loss. The absence of epidermis and dermis.

Granulation Tissue. The pink/red, moist tissue that contains new blood vessels, collagen, fibroblasts, and inflammatory cells, which fills an open, previously deep wound when it starts to heal.

Growth Factors. Proteins that affect the proliferation, movement, maturation, and biosynthetic activity of cells. For the purposes of this guideline, these are proteins that can be produced by living cells.

Handwashing. Handwashing is the cornerstone of any infection-control program. Handwashing should be of sufficient duration to remove the transient microbial flora (10 seconds of soap and friction, followed by rinsing with running water).

Healing. A dynamic process in which anatomical and functional integrity is restored. This process can be monitored and measured. For wounds of the skin, it involves repair of the dermis (granulation tissue formation) and epidermis (epithelialization). Healed wounds represent a spectrum of repair: They can be ideally healed (tissue regeneration), minimally healed (temporary return of anatomical continuity), or acceptably healed (sustained functional and anatomical result). The acceptably healed wound is the ultimate outcome of wound healing but not necessarily the appropriate outcome for all patients.

> **Primary Intention Healing.** Closure and healing of a sutured wound.
>
> **Secondary Intention Healing.** Closure and healing of a wound by the formation of granulation tissue and epithelialization.

Hydrotherapy. Use of whirlpool or submersion for wound cleansing.

Hypoalbuminemia. An abnormally low amount of albumin in the blood. A value less than 3.5 mg/dL is clinically significant. Albumin is the major serum protein that maintains plasma colloidal osmotic pressure (pressure within blood vessels) and transports fatty acids, bilirubin, and many drugs as well as certain hormones, such as cortisol and thyroxine, through the blood. Low serum albumin may be due to inadequate protein intake, active inflammation, or serious hepatic and renal disease and is associated with pressure ulcer development.

Infection. The presence of bacteria or other microorganisms in sufficient quantity to damage tissue or impair healing. Clinical experience has indicated that wounds can be classified as infected when the wound tissue contains 105 or greater microorganisms per gram of tissue. Clinical signs of infection may not be present, especially in the immunocompromised patient or the patient with a chronic wound.

Infection (Clinical). The presence of bacteria or other microorganisms in sufficient quantity to overwhelm the tissue defenses and produce the inflammatory signs of infection (i.e., purulent exudate, odor, erythema, warmth, tenderness, edema, pain, fever, and elevated white cell count).

> **Local Clinical Infection.** A clinical infection that is confined to the wound and within a few millimeters of its margins.
>
> **Systemic Clinical Infection.** A clinical infection that extends beyond the margins of the wound. Some systemic infectious complications of pressure ulcers include cellulitis, advancing cellulitis, osteomyelitis, meningitis, endocarditis, septic arthritis, bacteremia, and sepsis.

Inflammatory Response. A localized protective response elicited by injury or destruction of tissues that serves to destroy, dilute, or wall off both the injurious agent and the injured tissue. Clinical signs include pain, heat, redness, swelling, and loss of function. Inflammation may be diminished or absent in immunosuppressed patients.

Innervation. Nerve supply to an area of the body. Innervation is considered adequate if it is sufficient to sense temperature, touch, and pressure/pain and communicate this sensory information to the brain.

Intention. See Healing

Irrigation. Cleansing by a stream of fluid, preferably saline.

Ischemia. Deficiency of blood supply to a tissue, often leading to tissue necrosis.

Macerate. To soften by wetting or soaking. In this context, it refers to degenerative changes and disintegration of skin when it has been kept too moist.

Malnutrition. State of nutritional insufficiency due to either inadequate dietary intake or defective assimilation or utilization of food ingested. Clinically significant malnutrition is diagnosed if (1) serum albumin is less than 3.5 mg/dL, (2) the total lymphocyte count is less than 1,800/mm3, or (3) body weight has decreased more than 15 percent.

Necrotic Tissue. Tissue that has died and has therefore lost its usual physical properties and biological activity. Also called "devitalized tissue."

No-Touch Technique. Method of changing surface dressings without touching the wound or the surface of any dressing that may be in contact with the wound. Adherent dressings should be grasped by the corner and removed slowly, whereas gauze dressings can be pinched in the center and lifted off.

Osteomyelitis. An infectious inflammatory disease process in the bone that is often bacterial. One cost-effective method to determine osteomyelitis is to probe the wound with a sterile cotton-tipped application. If the tip can touch bone, osteomyelitis will be present in as many as 85% of the cases.

Pain. Nerve endings exposed to dressing removal and air can cause patients extreme discomfort. Moist wound healing is highly successful at reducing pain related to trauma of dressing removal.

Partial-Thickness Tissue Loss. Wounds that involve the epidermis and can extend into, but not through, the dermis. These wounds heal mainly by epithelialization, from the wound edges and from epithelial cells in the remaining hair follicles and glands.

Peri-Wound. The area surrounding the wound. Assessment of the edges may help to identify undermining (blue-gray or blanched), infection (erythema), or maceration (white margins).

Pressure (Interface). Force per unit area that acts perpendicularly to the body from the support surface. This parameter is affected by the stiffness of the support surface, the composition of the body tissue, and the geometry of the body being supported.

Pressure Reduction. Reduction of interface pressure, not necessarily below the level required to close capillaries (i.e., capillary-closing pressure).

Pressure Relief. Reduction of interface pressure below capillary-closing pressure.

Pressure Ulcer. Any lesion caused by unrelieved pressure resulting in damage of underlying tissue. They are also called decubitus ulcers, pressure sores, or bedsores. They are usually located over bony prominences and are graded or staged to classify the degree of tissue damage observed.

psi. Pounds per square inch—a unit of pressure; in this case, the pressure exerted by a stream of fluid against 1 square inch of skin or wound surface.

Purulent Discharge/Drainage. A product of inflammation that contains pus—i.e., cells (leukocytes, bacteria) and liquified necrotic debris.

Reactive Hyperemia. Reddening of the skin caused by blood rushing back into ischemic tissue.

Repositioning. Any change in body position that relieves pressure from tissue overlying bony prominences. Periodic repositioning of chairbound and bedfast individuals is one of the most basic and frequently used methods of reducing pressure. The overall goal of respositioning is to allow tissue reperfusion and thus prevent ischemic tissue changes. The term "repositioning" implies a sustained relief of pressure, not just a temporary shift. Specific repositioning techniques and the frequency of repositioning should be individualized according to the patient's level of risk and the goals of care.

Sepsis. The presence of various pus-forming and other pathogenic organisms or their toxins in the blood or tissues. Clinical signs of bloodborne sepsis include fever, tachycardia, hypotension, leukocytosis, and a deterioration in mental status. The same organism is often isolated in both the blood and the pressure ulcer.

Shear. Mechanical force that acts on a unit area of skin in a direction parallel to the body's surface. Shear is affected by the amount of pressure exerted, the coefficient of friction between the materials contacting each other, and the extent to which the body makes contact with the support surface.

Sinus Tract. A cavity or channel underlying a wound that involves an area larger than the visible surface of the wound.

Slough. Necrotic (dead) tissue in the process of separating from viable portions of the body.

Stasis Ulcer. Ulceration associated with ambulatory venous hypertension.

Support Surfaces. Special beds, mattresses, mattress overlays, or seat cushions that reduce or relieve pressure while sitting or lying.

Surfactants. A surface-active agent that reduces the surface tension of fluids to allow greater penetration.

Topical Antibiotic. A drug known to inhibit or kill microorganisms that can be applied locally to a tissue surface.

Topical Antiseptic. Product with antimicrobial activity designed for use on skin or other superficial tissues; may damage some cells.

Trochanter. Bony prominence on the upper part of the femur.

Tunneling. A passageway under the surface of the skin that is generally open at the skin level; however, most of the tunneling is not visible.

Underlying Tissue. Tissue that lies beneath the surface of the skin such as fatty tissue, supporting structures, muscle, and bone.

Undermining. A closed passageway under the surface of the skin that is open only at the skin surface. Generally it appears as an area of skin ulceration at the margins of the ulcer with skin overlying the area. Undermining often develops from shearing forces.

Quick Assessment of Leg Ulcers

	Venous Insufficiency (Stasis)	Arterial Insufficiency	Peripheral Neuropathy
History	Previous DVT and varicosities Reduced mobility Obesity Vascular ulcers Phlebitis Traumatic injury CHF Orthopaedic procedures Pain reduced by elevation	Diabetes Anemia Arthritis Increased pain with activity and/or elevation CVA Smoking Intermittent claudication Traumatic injury to extremity Vascular procedures/surgeries Hypertension Hyperlipidemia Arterial disease	Diabetes Spinal cord injury Hansen's disease Relief of pain with ambulation Paresthesia of extremities
Location	Medial aspect of lower leg and ankle Superior to medial malleolus	Toetips or web spaces Phalangeal heads around lateral malleolus Areas exposed to pressure or repetitive trauma	Plantar aspect of foot Metatarsal heads Heels Altered pressure points/sites of painless trauma/repetitive stress
Appearance	Color: base ruddy Surrounding skin: erythema (venous dermatitis) and/or brown staining (hyperpigmentation) Depth: usually shallow Wound margins: irregular Exudate: moderate to heavy Edema: pitting or nonpitting; possible induration and cellulitis Skin temp: normal; warm to touch Granulation: frequently present Infection: less common	Color: base of wound, pale/pallor on elevation; dependent rubor Skin: shiny, taut, thin, dry, hair loss on lower extremities, atrophy of subcutaneous tissue Depth: deep Wound margins: even Exudate: minimal Edema: variable Skin temp: decreased/cold Granulation tissue: rarely present Infection: frequent (signs may be subtle) Necrosis, eschar, gangrene may be present	Color: normal skin tones; trophic skin changes, fissuring and/or callus formation Depth: variable Wound margins: well defined Exudate: variable Edema: cellulitis, erythema, and induration common Skin temp: warm Granulation tissue: frequently present Infection: frequent Necrotic tissue variable, gangrene uncommon Reflexes usually diminished Altered gait; orthopaedic deformities common

Perfusion	Pain	Pain	Pain
	• Minimal unless infected or desiccated	• Intermittent claudication	• Diminished sensitivity to touch
	Peripheral pulses	• Resting	• Reduced response to pin prick, usually painless
	• Present/palpable	• Positional	Peripheral pulses
	Capillary refill	• Nocturnal	• Palpable/present
	• Normal—less than 3 seconds	Peripheral pulses	Capillary refill
		• Absent or diminished	• Normal
		Capillary refill	
		• Delayed—more than 3 seconds	
		• ABI < 0.8	
	Measures to improve venous return	Measures to improve tissue perfusion	Measures to eliminate trauma
	• Surgical obliteration of damaged veins	• Revascularization if possible	• Pressure relief for heel ulcers
	• Elevation of legs	• Medications to improve red blood cell transit through narrowed vessels	• "Offloading" for plantar ulcers (bedfast or contact casting or orthopaedic shoes)
	• Compression therapy to provide at least 30 mm Hg compression at ankle, using	• Lifestyle changes (no tobacco, no caffeine, no constrictive garments, avoidance of cold)	• Appropriate footwear
	• Short stretch bandages (e.g., Setopress, Surepress, Comprilan)	• Hydration	Tight glucose control
	• Therapeutic support stockings	• Measures to prevent trauma to tissues (appropriate footwear at all times)	Aggressive infection control (debridement of any necrotic tissue, orthopaedic consult for exposed bone, antibiotic coverage)
	• Unna Boot	Topical therapy	Topical therapy
	• Profore 4-layer wrap	• Dry uninfected necrotic wound; keep dry	• Cautious use of occlusive dressings
	• Compression pumps	• Dry infected wound, immediate referral for surgical debridement/aggressive antibiotic therapy	• Dressings to absorb exudate/keep surface moist
	Topical therapy	• Open wound	
	• Goals: absorb exudate, maintain moist wound surface (e.g., alginate, foam, hydrocolloid dressings)	• Moist wound healing	
		• Nonocclusive dressings (e.g., solid hydrogels) or cautious use of occlusive dressings	
		• Aggressive treatment of any infection	

SOURCES

CHAPTER 2

Figure 2–3 Courtesy of Knoll Pharmaceuticals, 1999, Mount Olive, New Jersey.

Table 2–1 Reprinted from B.M. Bates-Jensen, Management of Exudate and Infection, in *Wound Care: A Collaborative Practice Manual for Physical Therapists and Nurses*, C. Sussman, B.M. Bates-Jensen, eds., p. 160, (c) 1998, Aspen Publishers, Inc.

CHAPTER 3

Figure 3–1 Courtesy of Knoll Pharmaceuticals, 1999, Mount Olive, New Jersey.

Table 3–1 Reprinted from C. Sussman, Assessment of the Skin and Wound, in *Wound Care: A Collaborative Practice Manual for Physical Therapists and Nurses*, C. Sussman, B.M. Bates-Jensen, eds., p. 54, (c) 1998, Aspen Publishers, Inc.

CHAPTER 4

Exhibit 4–1 Courtesy of Ross Products Division of Abbott Laboratories, 2000, Columbus, Ohio.

Exhibit 4–2 Courtesy of Healthcare Dietary Services, Inc., 1999, Evansville, Indiana.

Exhibit 4–3 Courtesy of Healthcare Dietary Services, Inc., 1999, Evansville, Indiana.

Exhibit 4–4 Courtesy of Kaiser Permanente, Southern California Regional Health Education, 1999, Los Robles, California.

Exhibit 4–5 Courtesy of Healthcare Dietary Services, Inc., 1999, Evansville, Indiana.

CHAPTER 5

CHAPTER 6

Exhibit 6–1 Courtesy of the National Pressure Ulcer Advisory Panel, 2000, Reston, Virginia.

Exhibit 6–2 Copyright (c) 1988, Barbara J. Braden and Nancy Bergstrom.

Exhibit 6–3 Courtesy of Ross Products Division of Abbott Laboratories Inc., 1999, Columbus, Ohio.

Exhibit 6–5 Reprinted from B.M. Bates-Jensen, Pressure Ulcers: Pathophysiology and Prevention, in *Wound Care: A Collaborative Practice Manual for Physical Therapists and Nurses,* C. Sussman, B.M. Bates-Jensen, eds., pp. 267–268, (c) 1998, Aspen Publishers, Inc.

CHAPTER 7

Appendix 7–A Courtesy of Curative Health Service, 2000, Hauppauge, New York.

CHAPTER 8

Exhibit 8–1 Adapted from L.A. Wiersema-Bryant, Management of Edema, in *Wound Care: A Collaborative Practice Manual for Physical Therapists and Nurses,* C. Sussman, B.M. Bates-Jensen, eds., pp. 180–198, (c) 1998, Aspen Publishers, Inc.

Exhibit 8–2 Adapted from L.A. Wiersema-Bryant, Management of Edema, in *Wound Care: A Collaborative Practice Manual for Physical Therapists and Nurses,* C. Sussman, B.M. Bates-Jensen, eds., pp. 185–186, (c) 1998, Aspen Publishers, Inc.

Exhibit 8–3 Courtesy of Curative Health Service, 2000, Hauppauge, New York.

Table 8–1 Adapted from L.A. Wiersema-Bryant, Management of Edema, in *Wound Care: A Collaborative Practice Manual for Physical Therapists and Nurses,* C. Sussman, B.M. Bates-Jensen, eds., p. 181, (c) 1998, Aspen Publishers, Inc.

CHAPTER 10

Exhibit 10–1 Reprinted with permission from F.E.W. Wagner, the Wagner Scale from *The Dysvascular Foot: A System for Diagnosis and Treatment, Foot and Ankle,* Vol. 2, pp. 64–122, (c) 1981, Williams & Wilkins.

Exhibit 10–2 Reprinted with permission from J.C. Duffy and C.A. Patout, Figure 1 of Management of the Insensitive Foot in Diabetes, *Military Medicine: International Journal of AMSUS,* Vol. 155, No. 12, p. 575, (c) 1990, Association of Military Surgeons of the United States, The Society of the Federal Health Agencies.

Exhibit 10–3 Adapted from *Feet Can Last a Lifetime,* National Institute of Diabetes and Digestive and Kidney Diseases, U.S. Department of Health and Human Services, National Institutes of Health, November, 1997, Bethesda, Maryland.

Exhibit 10–4 Reprinted with permission from J.C. Duffy and C.A. Patout, Figure 1 of Management of the Insensitive Foot in Diabetes, *Military Medicine: International Journal of AMSUS,* Vol. 155, No. 12, p. 575, (c) 1990, Association of Military Surgeons of the United States, The Society of the Federal Health Agencies.

Exhibit 10–5 Courtesy of Curative Health Service, 2000, Hauppauge, New York.

Figure 10–1 Reprinted from N. Elftman, Management of the Neuropathic Foot, in *Wound Care: A Collaborative Practice Manual for Physical Therapists and Nurses,* C. Sussman, B.M. Bates-Jensen, eds., p. 331, (c) 1998, Aspen Publishers, Inc.

Figure 10–5 Reprinted from N. Elftman, Management of the Neuropathic Foot, in *Wound Care: A Collaborative Practice Manual for Physical Therapists and Nurses,* C. Sussman, B.M. Bates-Jensen, eds., p. 336, (c) 1998, Aspen Publishers, Inc.

CHAPTER 12

Exhibit 12–1 Reprinted from B.M. Bates-Jensen and J. Wethe, Acute Surgical Wound Management, in *Wound Care: A Collaborative Practice Manual for Physical Therapists and Nurses,* C. Sussman and B. Bates-Jensen, eds., p. 232, (c) 1998, Aspen Publishers, Inc.

Exhibit 12–2 Courtesy of Coloplast Corporation, 2000, Marietta, Georgia.

Table 12–1 Reprinted from B.M. Bates-Jensen and J. Wethe, Acute Surgical Wound Management, in *Wound Care: A Collaborative Practice Manual for Physical Therapists and Nurses,* C. Sussman and B. Bates-Jensen, eds., p. 229, (c) 1998, Aspen Publishers, Inc.

Table 12–2 Reprinted from B.M. Bates-Jensen and J. Wethe, Acute Surgical Wound Management, in *Wound Care: A Collaborative Practice Manual for Physical Therapists and Nurses,* C. Sussman and B. Bates-Jensen, eds., p. 230, (c) 1998, Aspen Publishers, Inc.

CHAPTER 13

Exhibit 13–1 Reprinted from the Health Care Financing Administration, Department of Health and Human Services.

Exhibit 13–2 Reprinted from the Health Care Financing Administration, Department of Health and Human Services.

CHAPTER 14

Exhibit 14–1 Reprinted from the Health Care Financing Administration, Department of Health and Human Services.

Exhibit 14–2 Reprinted from the Health Care Financing Administration, Department of Health and Human Services.

GLOSSARY

Adapted from *AHCPR Treatment Guidelines #15*, Agency for Healthcare Policy and Research, U.S. Department of Health and Human Services, Rockville, Maryland, 1994.

APPENDIX A

Courtesy of Wound, Ostomy and Continence Nurses Society, 1999, Costa Mesa, California.

INDEX